GASTRITIS DIET COOKBOOK FOR BEGINNERS

Journey through a day of gastritis-friendly meals, starting with nourishing breakfasts and ending with satisfying dinners, ensuring every bite contributes to your well-being.

SMART DESTY

Table of Contents

INTRODUCTION

Gastritis is a prevalent digestive condition that affects millions of individuals throughout the world, reducing their quality of life and general well-being. As a well-trained nutritionist, you must dig into the complexities of gastritis, including its nature, causes, symptoms, and the critical role that a gastritis-friendly diet plays in controlling and avoiding the illness.

What is Gastritis?

Gastritis is inflammation of the stomach lining, which can be moderate or severe. The stomach lining is an important part of the digestive system because it produces stomach acids and enzymes that help the body break down food. When the lining becomes inflamed, it can cause irritation, pain, and, in extreme situations, problems.

Gastritis inflammation can be acute, meaning it occurs quickly and lasts just a short time, or chronic, meaning it lasts for a long time. Acute gastritis is commonly caused by irritants such as alcohol, certain medicines, or infections, but chronic gastritis can be caused by long-term irritants such as Helicobacter pylori (H. pylori) infection, autoimmune diseases, or extended use of nonsteroidal anti-inflammatory drugs (NSAIDs).

Causes and Symptoms

Understanding the causes of gastritis is critical to successful prevention and treatment. As previously stated, acute gastritis can be caused by excessive alcohol intake, extended use of NSAIDs, bacterial infections, or stress. Chronic gastritis, on the other hand, is frequently linked to chronic H. pylori infection, autoimmune illnesses, or other underlying health issues.

Gastritis symptoms can vary, but frequent ones include stomach discomfort, bloating, nausea, vomiting, indigestion, and a sense of fullness. In more severe situations, gastritis can cause bleeding and stomach ulcers.

Identifying the underlying cause of gastritis is critical for personalized treatment, which frequently necessitates contact with healthcare specialists. Once the reason is identified, a multimodal strategy, including dietary changes, becomes an essential component in properly managing gastritis.

Benefits of a Gastritis-Friendly Diet:

A well-planned diet can help manage gastritis symptoms and promote recovery. A gastritis-friendly diet seeks to soothe the stomach lining, relieve symptoms, and promote overall digestive health. Nutrient-rich, stomach-friendly meals can help avoid gastritis flare-ups and speed up the healing process.

A gastritis-friendly diet is important since it can treat several facets of the ailment. It aids in inflammation management, stomach acid reduction, irritation prevention, and support for the body's natural healing processes. A balanced diet also promotes general digestive health, which is essential for preventing gastritis recurrence and preserving long-term well-being.

Developing a Gastritis-Friendly Diet:

Designing a gastritis-friendly diet necessitates a thorough and personalized approach, as each person's tolerance for certain foods varies. However, there are broad suggestions that may be used as a foundation for developing a diet that supports gastritis management:

Promote Whole, Nutrient-Rich Foods:

Whole, nutrient-dense meals are crucial for giving the body with the vitamins and minerals it needs to recover. A diet that is good for gastritis should include fresh fruits and vegetables, lean meats, whole grains, and healthy fats. These meals not only provide necessary nutrients, but they are also gentler on the stomach, lowering the chance of inflammation.

Limit or avoid irritant foods.

Certain meals and beverages might worsen gastritis symptoms by irritating the stomach lining. Spicy meals, acidic fruits, caffeine, alcohol, and fatty foods are all common causes that should be reduced or avoided. These chemicals can raise stomach acid levels or induce inflammation, impeding the healing process.

Small and Frequent Meals:

Individuals with gastritis may benefit from eating smaller, more frequent meals rather than larger ones. This method helps to avoid placing too much load on the digestive system, reducing pain and facilitating better digestion. Eating slowly and carefully can improve the digestive process while lowering the chance of symptom aggravation

Hydration is Key:

Adequate hydration is necessary for general health, but it is especially important for people who have gastritis. Water promotes mucosal integrity and aids the digestion process. However, carbonated beverages, particularly those with high acidity, should be minimized since they might cause gastrointestinal discomfort.

Probiotics for Gut Health:

Probiotics, which are commonly present in fermented foods such as yogurt, kefir, and sauerkraut, can help promote intestinal health. These "friendly" bacteria help to maintain a healthy microbiome, which is necessary for proper digestion. However, probiotics should be introduced cautiously since some people with gastritis are sensitive to fermented foods.

Individualised Approach:

While these broad principles provide a good basis, it is critical to understand the unique characteristics of gastritis and modify dietary advice appropriately. Some people can tolerate meals that others cannot. Keeping a food diary and documenting how the body reacts to different meals might be useful in tailoring a gastritis-friendly diet.

CHAPTER ONE: GETTING STARTED

Gastritis is a disorder that demands careful and meticulous management. This chapter seeks to help people in the early stages of controlling gastritis by covering important topics including diagnosis, healthcare professional consultation, and setting realistic dietary objectives.

Diagnosing Gastritis

Before making any dietary changes, it is critical to have a precise diagnosis of gastritis. Gastritis is diagnosed after a comprehensive review of the patient's medical history, a physical examination, and, in many cases, specialist testing. Gastroscopy, which involves inserting a flexible tube with a camera into the mouth to inspect the stomach lining, is a popular diagnostic technique.

Blood tests may also be performed to determine the existence of H. pylori infection or other underlying reasons. A clear diagnosis allows healthcare personnel to personalize therapies according on the type and severity of gastritis, setting the groundwork for a successful management strategy.

As a nutritionist, it is critical to work with healthcare specialists during the diagnosis process. This partnership guarantees that dietary advice are appropriate for the recognized cause and severity of gastritis, supporting a comprehensive and individualized approach to care.

Consult with a Healthcare Professional
A consultation with a healthcare practitioner is an important step in the process of controlling gastritis. Gastroenterologists, primary care doctors, and nutritionists that specialize in digestive health can offer helpful insights and advice. These specialists may assist in interpreting diagnostic data, identifying relevant variables, and developing a complete management strategy.

Individuals suffering with gastritis should be candid about their symptoms, eating habits, and lifestyle variables throughout their appointment. This information helps healthcare practitioners adjust interventions to each individual's specific requirements and circumstances. Collaboration with healthcare specialists also ensures that any underlying disorders causing gastritis are treated, resulting in a more comprehensive and successful management strategy.

As a nutritionist, regularly communicating with healthcare providers enables the smooth integration of nutritional solutions into the entire treatment plan. This partnership improves the efficacy of therapies and ensures that dietary suggestions complement medical interventions for the best results.

Developing Realistic Dietary Goals
Setting realistic dietary goals is an essential part of controlling gastritis. It entails making manageable and sustained modifications to one's dietary habits that promote digestive health and relieve symptoms. The key to defining realistic dietary objectives is to consider individual tastes, lifestyle circumstances, and the severity of gastritis.

Personal preferences must be considered in order to guarantee compliance with the necessary dietary adjustments. Individuals are more likely to stick with dietary changes that are consistent with their likes and preferences. Furthermore, the degree of gastritis influences the extent of dietary restrictions required. For example, people with acute gastritis may require more rigorous dietary modifications at first, but those with chronic gastritis may focus on long-term dietary habits.

A nutritionist, in partnership with other healthcare specialists, can assist clients in setting dietary objectives that are particular to their situation. This includes teaching people about gastritis-friendly foods, supporting them to make educated decisions, and offering practical advice for incorporating these changes into their everyday life.

Setting realistic dietary goals requires considering not just which foods to include or avoid, but also how to develop a balanced and satisfying eating habit. This fosters a good relationship with food and facilitates long-term adherence to prescribed dietary adjustments.

Dietary choices have a considerable impact on the treatment of gastritis. This chapter delves into the foundations of a gastritis-friendly diet, providing an overview of essential ideas, particular items to include, and those to avoid.

Gastritis-Friendly Diet

A gastritis diet focuses on minimizing stomach lining irritation, relieving symptoms, and promoting recovery. The main ideas include eating nutrient-dense, readily digested meals that improve gastric health. This nutritional strategy emphasizes macronutrient balance, healthy foods, and individual tolerances.

This diet not only helps to manage symptoms but also promotes overall digestive health. It seeks to reduce elements that contribute to inflammation and pain, hence enabling stomach lining healing.

Foods To Include
Alkaline foods:
Alkaline foods are a key component of a gastritis-friendly diet. Alkaline meals assist to neutralize stomach acid, lowering the risk of discomfort. Fruits like bananas, melons, and apples are alkaline and easy on the stomach. Vegetables like spinach, kale, and cucumber are all wonderful options.

Whole grains, such as oats and quinoa, as well as nuts and seeds, help to keep the body alkaline. Alkaline water can also be used to help with hydration and pH balance.

High Fiber Options:
Fiber-rich meals are essential for good digestive health. They stimulate regular bowel motions and help with overall gut health. Choosing whole grains, such as brown rice and whole wheat, promotes enough fiber consumption. Legumes, like lentils and chickpeas, are high in fiber and include plant-based protein.

Fruits and vegetables high in fiber, such as broccoli, carrots, and berries, are healthy additions to a gastritis diet. The soluble fiber in oats and flaxseeds can help maintain digestive regularity without putting too much strain on the stomach.

Foods To Avoid

Trigger foods:

Identifying and avoiding trigger foods is essential for treating gastritis symptoms. Trigger foods are ones that can worsen inflammation, raise stomach acid levels, or create discomfort. Fried and fatty meals, as well as processed foods with high levels of chemicals and preservatives, are common triggers.

Individual sensitivities vary, but frequent trigger foods include some dairy products, especially those high in fat. Individuals must pay attention to how their bodies respond to certain foods and avoid or restrict those that cause gastritis symptoms.

Acidic and spicy foods:

Acidic and spicy meals might aggravate gastritis symptoms due to their irritating properties. Citrus fruits, tomatoes, and citrus liquids are acidic, which may cause pain. Spices such as chile, pepper, and spicy sauce can also aggravate inflammation and should be used carefully or avoided.

Carbonated drinks, such as sodas, are acidic and can cause bloating and gas. Caffeine, present in coffee and other teas, can increase stomach acid production, thereby exacerbating gastritis symptoms. Choosing non-acidic alternatives and decaffeinated ones might be advantageous.

CHAPTER 3: BREAKFAST RECIPES.

Recipe 1: Banana Almond Smoothie Bowl.

This energetic Banana Almond Smoothie Bowl is a delicious and relaxing way to begin the day. This meal, packed with potassium from bananas and the healthy flavor of almonds, is not only easy on the stomach but also high in critical minerals. It's an excellent alternative for individuals on a gastritis-friendly diet.

Ingredient list:
- two ripe bananas, peeled and frozen
- 1/4 cup almond butter.
- 1 cup unsweetened almond milk
- 1 tablespoon chia seeds.
- -1/4 cup rolled oats
- Toppings include sliced almonds, fresh berries, and a drizzle of honey.

Two servings.

Instructions:
1. Blend frozen bananas, almond butter, almond milk, chia seeds, and rolled oats.
2. Blend until smooth and creamy.
3. Pour the smoothie into bowls and garnish with sliced almonds, fresh berries, and honey.
4. Serve immediately and savor this nutritious and calming breakfast.

Notes, Features, and Variations:
- Add plain, low-fat Greek yogurt for extra protein.
- To add variation, customize the toppings with your favorite fruits and nuts.
- To adjust the thickness of the smoothie, add more or less almond milk according to personal desire.

Utensils needed include a blender, serving dishes, and measuring cups.

Nutritional information:

Per serving: 250 calories, 7g protein, 12g fat, 30g carbs, and 6g fiber.

Recipe #2: Quinoa Breakfast Bowl

Begin the day with this nutrient-dense Quinoa Breakfast Bowl. Quinoa, known for its high protein and fiber content, is combined with fresh fruits and a touch of honey to make a filling and stomach-friendly breakfast. This formula delivers long-lasting energy and helps intestinal health.

Ingredients:

- 1 cup cooked quinoa,
- 1/2 cup unsweetened almond milk.
- 1/2 teaspoon of ground cinnamon.
- 1 tablespoon honey,
- 1/2 cup mixed fresh berries,
- 1 tablespoon chopped nuts (walnuts or almonds).

Two servings.

Instructions:

1. Warm cooked quinoa in a pot with almond milk over medium heat.
2. Stir in the ground cinnamon and honey until well blended.
3. Separate the quinoa mixture into bowls.
4. Top each bowl with a combination of fresh berries and chopped almonds.
5. Drizzle with more honey if desired.
6. Serve warm and enjoy this nutritious, gastritis-friendly breakfast.

Notes, Features, and Variations:

- Experiment with various fruits and nuts to create unique flavor profiles.
- Before serving, add a dollop of coconut yogurt for an extra creamy texture.
- To adjust the sweetness, change the amount of honey to your liking.

Utensils needed are a saucepan, stirring spoon, and serving dishes.

Nutritional information:

Per serving: 280 calories, 8g protein, 6g fat, 50g carbohydrates, and 7g fiber.

Recipe #3: Blueberry Oat Pancakes

These Blueberry Oat Pancakes are a delicious variation on a traditional breakfast staple. This dish, which includes oats and antioxidant-rich blueberries, is easy on the stomach and improves digestive comfort. You may enjoy a stack of these fluffy pancakes without feeling guilty.

Ingredients:

- 1 cup rolled oats,
- 1/2 cup unsweetened almond milk,
- 1 ripe banana.
- Half cup fresh or frozen blueberries
- One teaspoon of baking powder.
- 1/2 teaspoon of vanilla essence.
- Coconut oil for cooking.

Two servings.

Instructions

1: In a blender, mix rolled oats, almond milk, banana, baking powder, and vanilla extract.
2. Blend until a smooth batter is formed.
3. Gently mix the blueberries into the batter.
4. Heat the coconut oil in a nonstick pan over medium heat.
5. Pour 1/4 cup of batter onto the pan to make pancakes.
6. Cook until bubbles appear on the surface, then turn and cook the opposite side.
7. Serve warm and enjoy these fluffy, gastritis-friendly pancakes.

Notes, Features, and Variations:

- Replace blueberries with low-acid fruits such as sliced strawberries or chopped apples.
- Add a spoonful of coconut whipped cream for extra enjoyment.
- If desired, adjust the sweetness with a small amount of maple syrup.

Utensils required: blender, nonstick pan, and spatula.

Nutritional information:

Per serving: 320 calories, 7g protein, 8g fat, 55g carbs, and 8g fiber.

Recipe 4: Avocado toast with poached egg.

Avocado toast with poached egg is a flavorful and filling breakfast choice that is easy on the stomach. Avocado's creamy texture complements the protein-packed poached egg, making for a nutrient-dense and gastritis-friendly lunch. This dish is quick, simple, and ideal for hectic mornings.

Ingredient list:

- 2 slices whole grain bread, toasted
- One ripe avocado, mashed
- Two poached eggs
- Season with salt and pepper as desired.
- Optional toppings. Fresh herbs and chili flakes.

Two servings.

Instructions:

1. Toast whole grain bread to desired crispiness.
2. Spread the mashed avocado evenly across each slice.
3. Top each piece with a poached egg.
4. Add salt and pepper to taste.
5. Optional garnishes include fresh herbs and chili flakes.
6. Serve immediately for a nutritious and flavorful breakfast.

Notes, Features, and Variations:

- Optional toppings include sliced tomatoes and nutritional yeast.
- Experiment with different kinds of bread, such sourdough or gluten-free alternatives.
- Drizzle with olive oil just before serving for an extra creamy texture.

Utensils required: toaster, poaching pan, and spreading knife.

Nutritional information:

Per serving: 280 calories, 12g protein, 15g fat, 25g carbs, and 8g fiber.

Recipe #5: Chia Seed Pudding with Mango

Enjoy a lovely Chia Seed Pudding with Mango for a breakfast that is both soft on the stomach and decadently delicious. Chia seeds include omega-3 fatty acids and fiber, while ripe mango adds natural sweetness. This meal not only tastes good, but it also helps with digestion.

Ingredients:

- 1/4 cup chia seeds.
- 1 cup unsweetened almond milk
- 1 tablespoon maple syrup.
- 1/2 teaspoon vanilla essence,
- 1 diced mango, and sliced almonds for garnish.

Two servings.

Procedure:

1. In a dish, mix the chia seeds, almond milk, maple syrup, and vanilla extract.
2. Stir thoroughly and set aside for 5 minutes.
3. Stir the mixture again to avoid clumping, then chill for at least 2 hours or overnight.
4. To serve, top the chia pudding with chopped mango in serving glasses.
5. Add sliced almonds for crunch.
6. Enjoy this nutrient-dense Chia Seed Pudding with Mango.

Notes, Features, and Variations:

- Try alternative fruit combinations, such berries or kiwi.
- Before refrigerating the chia pudding, combine it to enhance smoothness.
- To adjust the sweetness, change the amount of maple syrup to your liking.

Utensils needed are a mixing bowl, stirring spoon, and serving glasses.

Nutritional information:

Per serving: 220 calories, 5g protein, 10g fat, 30g carbs, and 10g fiber.

Recipe #6: Spinach and Feta Omelet

This Spinach and Feta Omelette is a flavorful, protein-rich breakfast option that is easy on the stomach. Spinach has important nutrients, while feta adds taste. This quick and simple dish is ideal for a tasty and gastritis-friendly breakfast.

Ingredients:

- 3 big eggs.
- 1 cup chopped fresh spinach
- 1/4 cup crumbled feta cheese.
- Season with salt and pepper to taste.
- 1 teaspoon olive oil.

Two servings.

Procedure:

1. In a mixing basin, whisk together the eggs until thoroughly combined.
2. Heat the olive oil in a nonstick pan over medium heat.
3. Add the chopped spinach to the pan and cook until wilted.
4. Pour beaten eggs over the spinach and allow it set slightly.
5. Sprinkle crumbled feta equally over one half of the omelette.
6. Fold the remaining half over the filling and heat until the eggs are well done.
7. Add salt and pepper to taste.
8. Serve warm for a tasty, gastritis-friendly breakfast.

Notes, Features, and Variations:

- Add chopped tomatoes or bell peppers for more flavor and nutrition.
- Try various herbs, such as dill or parsley, for extra freshness.
- For a kick, add your favorite low-acid hot sauce.

Utensils required: Whisk, nonstick pan, and spatula.

Nutritional information:

Per serving: 240 calories, 18g protein, 16g fat, 4g carbohydrates, and 1g fiber.

Recipe #7: Salmon and Avocado Wrap

The Salmon and Avocado Wrap is a filling and omega-3-rich breakfast choice that is gentle on the stomach. The combination of smoked salmon and creamy avocado creates a delicious taste profile, making this a nutritional and gastritis-friendly option.

Ingredient list:

- Two whole grain tortillas.
- Four ounces of smoked salmon
- 1 sliced avocado,
- 2 tablespoons unsweetened Greek yogurt, and fresh dill for garnish.

Two servings.

Procedure:

1. Spread Greek yogurt equally on the tortillas.
2. Arrange smoked salmon and avocado slices on the tortillas.
3. To enhance taste, garnish with fresh dill.
4. Roll the tortillas into wraps and cut in half.
5. Serve immediately for a quick and hearty breakfast.

Notes, Features, and Variations:

- Squeeze lemon for added brightness and vitamin C.
- Add a handful of leafy greens, such arugula or spinach, for extra benefits.
- Add a dash of black pepper for more taste.

Utensils needed: knife and chopping board.

Nutritional information:

Per serving: 280 calories, 18g protein, 16g fat, 22g carbohydrates, and 7g fiber.

Recipe #8: Sweet Potato Breakfast Hash

This Sweet Potato Breakfast Hash is a filling and nutritious meal that is gentle on the digestive system. Sweet potatoes are high in vitamins and minerals, making them an excellent basis for this tasty meal. When combined with eggs and veggies, it's a tasty and filling option.

Ingredients:

- 2 medium sweet potatoes, peeled and diced
- 1 tablespoon olive oil - Diced bell pepper
- 1 chopped onion and 2 eggs.
- Salt and pepper to taste.
- Garnish with fresh parsley.

Serves: 2

Procedure:

1. Heat olive oil in a pan over medium heat.
2. Add the diced sweet potatoes and sauté until golden brown and soft.
3. Add the diced bell pepper and onion to the pan and cook until softened.
4. Form two wells in the hash and crack an egg into each.
5. Cover the skillet and cook the eggs to your preference.
6. Add salt and pepper to taste.
7. Finish with fresh parsley and serve warm.

Notes, Features, and Variations:

- Add cherry tomatoes for a fresh taste.
- For added taste, sprinkle with feta or goat cheese.
- Add your preferred herbs, such as thyme or rosemary.

Utensils needed: Skillet and spatula.

Nutritional information:

Per serving: 320 calories, 10g protein, 12g fat, 45g carbs, and 7g fiber.

Recipe 9: Cucumber and Turkey Roll-ups

Cucumber and Turkey Roll-Ups are a delicious, protein-packed breakfast that is easy on the stomach. These roll-ups are not only easy to make, but they also have a delightful crunch and savory flavor. A great option for a light, gastritis-friendly breakfast.

Ingredients:

- One big cucumber, peeled into ribbons.

- 4 ounces of turkey breast slices.

- 1/4 cup hummus - Cherry tomatoes as garnish

- Fresh basil leaves as garnish

Two servings.

Procedure:

1. Spread a thin layer of hummus on cucumber ribbons.
2. Place turkey breast slices on the cucumber with hummus.
3. Roll up each cucumber ribbon with the turkey inside.
4. Secure with toothpicks if required.
5. Garnish with cherry tomatoes and fresh basil leaves.
6. Serve chilled for a refreshing, gastritis-friendly breakfast.

Notes, Features, and Variations:

- For more taste, sprinkle with ground black pepper or paprika.

- Experiment with different flavors of hummus, including roasted red pepper or garlic.

- Add avocado slices for extra richness.

Utensils needed: Peeler and toothpicks.

Nutritional information:

Per serving: 200 calories, 15g protein, 8g fat, 15g carbs, and 4g fiber.

Recipe #10: Greek Yogurt Parfait with Berries

Enjoy the creamy richness of a Greek Yogurt Parfait with Berries for a delicious and stomach-filling breakfast. This parfait blends the richness of Greek yogurt, the sweetness of fresh berries, and the crunch of oats. A simple but pleasant option for a gastritis-friendly start to the day.

Ingredients:

- 1 cup Greek yogurt (unsweetened).
- half cup mixed berries (strawberries, blueberries, raspberries)
- 1/4 cup granola (low in added sugar)
- One spoonful of honey (optional).

Two servings.

Procedure:

1. In serving glasses or bowls, layer Greek yogurt with mixed berries.
2. To add crunch, sprinkle granola over each layer.
3. Repeat the layers until the glasses are full.
4. Drizzle with honey if more sweetness is required.
5. Serve immediately for a tasty and nutritious breakfast.

Notes, Features, and Variations:

- Experiment with other fruit combinations, such mango and pineapple.
- For a healthy choice, use granola with less added sugars.
- Add a sprinkling of cinnamon for added taste.

Utensils required: Serving glasses or bowls.

Nutritional information:

Per serving: 250 calories, 15g protein, 8g fat, 30g carbs, and 4g fiber.

Recipe 11: Overnight Chia Seed Pudding with Mixed Berries.

Make this Overnight Chia Seed Pudding with Mixed Berries the night before for a quick and healthy breakfast. Chia seeds include fiber and omega-3 fatty acids, while mixed berries offer natural sweetness. This dish is not only pleasant on the stomach, but it also provides a quick and tasty breakfast.

Ingredient list:

- 1/4 cup chia seeds.

- 1 cup almond milk, unsweetened

- One spoonful of maple syrup.

- 1/2 teaspoon vanilla essence

- 1/2 cup mixed berries (strawberries, blueberries, raspberries).

Two servings.

Directions:

1. In a dish, combine chia seeds, almond milk, maple syrup, and vanilla essence.
2. Mix well and chill overnight or for at least 4 hours.
3. Before serving, stir the chia pudding and top with mixed berries.
4. Serve chilled for a refreshing and nutrient-dense breakfast.

Notes, Features, and Variations:

- Try alternative plant-based milks, such as coconut or oat milk.
- Finish with a spoonful of coconut yogurt for extra richness.
- Garnish with shredded coconut or chopped almonds.

Utensils needed are a mixing bowl, stirring spoon, and serving glasses.

Nutritional information:

Per serving: 220 calories, 5g protein, 10g fat, 30g carbs, and 10g fiber.

Recipe 12: Turkey and Vegetable Breakfast Wrap.

This Turkey and Veggie Breakfast Wrap is a delicious and protein-rich alternative for a full breakfast. Turkey offers lean protein, and a variety of colorful veggies provide taste and nutrients. Wrapped in a whole grain tortilla, it's a stomach-friendly option that provides a healthy start to the day.

Ingredients:

- Two whole grain tortillas.

- 4 oz. cooked turkey breast, sliced

- 1/2 cup baby spinach leaves.

- 1/4 cup halved cherry tomatoes

- 1/4 cup sliced cucumber.

- Two tablespoons of unsweetened Greek yogurt

Two servings.

Procedure:

1. Spread Greek yogurt equally on the tortillas.

2. Place the turkey slices, baby spinach, cherry tomatoes, and cucumber on the tortillas.

3. Roll each tortilla into a wrap.

4. Cut in half and serve immediately for a delicious and nutritious breakfast.

Notes, Features, and Variations:

- Add feta cheese for additional taste.

- Experiment with various veggies, such as bell peppers and shredded carrots.

- Serve with a dab of olive oil or balsamic vinegar.

Utensils needed: knife and chopping board.

Nutritional information:

Per serving: 300 calories, 20g protein, 10g fat, 35g carbs, and 6g fiber.

Recipe 13: Mango and Coconut Overnight Oatmeal

Mango and Coconut Overnight Oats provide a tropical twist. This make-ahead breakfast, packed with the health of oats, fresh mango, and coconut, is not only easy on the stomach but also provides a delicious burst of tastes. Prepare the night before for a stress-free morning.

Ingredients:

- 1/2 cup rolled oats,
- 1/2 cup unsweetened coconut milk,
- 1/2 cup chopped mango,
- 1 tablespoon shredded coconut,
- 1 tablespoon maple syrup.

Two servings.

Procedure:

1. Combine rolled oats and coconut milk in a jar or container.
2. Combine the chopped mango, shredded coconut, and maple syrup.
3. Stir thoroughly, cover, and chill overnight.
4. Before serving, mix the oats and top with more mango and coconut if preferred.
5. Serve chilled for a tropical-inspired, gastritis-friendly breakfast.

Notes, Features, and Variations:

- Experiment with various fruits, such as pineapple or kiwi.
- For a dairy-free option, use almond or soy milk.
- Adjust the amount of maple syrup to achieve your desired sweetness.

Utensils needed:

Jar or container, stirring spoon.

Nutritional composition:

Calories: 280 per serving, Protein: 6g, Fat: 10g, Carbohydrates: 40g, Fiber: 5g.

Recipe 14: Apple Cinnamon Quinoa Porridge.

Start your morning with the soothing warmth of Apple Cinnamon Quinoa Porridge. Quinoa, a protein-rich grain, complements the natural sweetness of apples and the warmth of cinnamon. This hearty and filling porridge is an excellent choice for a healthful breakfast.

Ingredient list:

- 1/2 cup washed quinoa.
- 1 cup unsweetened almond milk,
- 1 peeled and chopped apple,
- 1/2 teaspoon ground cinnamon.
- 1 tablespoon of chopped walnuts (optional).
- one tablespoon maple syrup (optional)

Two servings.

Steps

1. In a saucepan, mix quinoa and almond milk.
2. Bring to a boil, then decrease heat to low, cover, and let simmer for 15 minutes.
3. Add the diced apple and ground cinnamon, stirring thoroughly.
4. Continue to boil until the quinoa is cooked and the apple is soft.
5. Divide the porridge across bowls, sprinkle with chopped walnuts, and drizzle with maple syrup if preferred.
6. Serve warm for a satisfying and gastritis-friendly breakfast.

Notes, Features, and Variations:

- Experiment with different apple kinds to adjust sweetness.
- Add a sprinkle of nutmeg for an added burst of flavour.
- Add a sprinkle of ground flaxseed for extra nutritious benefits.

Utensils required: Saucepan and stirring spoon.

Nutritional information:

Per serving: 300 calories, 8g protein, 8g fat, 50g carbohydrates, and 7g fiber.

Recipe 15: Blueberry Coconut Chia Popsicles.

Blueberry Coconut Chia Popsicles are a pleasant twist on breakfast. These popsicles, packed with the nutritious richness of chia seeds, coconut milk, and antioxidant-rich blueberries, are a refreshing and delicious treat that is easy on the stomach. Prepare them ahead of time for a fun, gastritis-friendly breakfast.

Ingredients:

-1/4 cup chia seeds.

- One cup unsweetened coconut milk.

- Half cup fresh or frozen blueberries

- 1 Tbsp honey - Popsicle molds

4 servings.

Instructions:

1. In a dish, combine chia seeds, coconut milk, blueberries, and honey.
2. Allow the mixture to settle for 10 minutes so that the chia seeds may expand.
3. Pour the mixture into the popsicle molds.
4. Freeze for at least four hours, or until completely set.
5. Once frozen, take the popsicles out of the molds and enjoy this novel and gastritis-friendly breakfast.

Notes, Features, and Variations:

- Experiment with different berries, such as raspberries and blackberries.
- Add a squeeze of lime juice for a punch of zesty flavor.
- Adjust the amount of honey to achieve your desired sweetness.

Utensils needed: Mixing bowl and popsicle molds.

Nutritional information:

Per serving: 120 calories, 3g protein, 8g fat, 15g carbs, and 5g fiber.

Recipe 16: Almond Butter and Banana Breakfast Quesadilla.

For a delicious and nutritious breakfast, try the Almond Butter and Banana Breakfast Quesadilla. This dish mixes the creamy texture of almond butter with the natural sweetness of bananas, all wrapped in a whole grain tortilla. A quick and tasty breakfast choice that is easy on the stomach.

Ingredients:

- Two whole grain tortillas.
- 4 tablespoons almond butter,
- 2 thinly sliced bananas,
- 1 tablespoon chia seeds (optional).
- One teaspoon of honey (optional)

Two servings.

Steps

1. Spread almond butter equally on each tortilla.
2. Place banana slices on one side of each tortilla.
3. Sprinkle chia seeds over the bananas.
4. Fold the tortillas in half to make quesadillas.
5. Cook in a skillet over medium heat until both sides are lightly browned.
6. Drizzle with honey if preferred.
7. Serve warm and enjoy this wonderful, gastritis-friendly breakfast.

Notes, Features, and Variations:

- Add a sprinkling of cinnamon for more taste.
- To make it nut-free, substitute sunflower seed butter for almond butter.
- Try different nut or seed toppings to provide variation.

Utensils needed: pan and spatula.

Nutritional information:

Per serving: 350 calories, 8g protein, 18g fat, 45g carbohydrates, and 7g fiber.

Recipe 17: Turmeric and Ginger Smoothie.

This Turmeric and Ginger Smoothie has anti-inflammatory effects that will help you start your day off well. Turmeric and ginger are a potent combination of health benefits, and when combined with fruits, they provide a refreshing and gastritis-friendly breakfast choice that promotes digestive health.

Ingredient list:

- One cup of frozen pineapple pieces
- One-half teaspoon turmeric powder
- 1/2 teaspoon fresh ginger, shredded
- One banana.
- One cup unsweetened coconut water.
- One spoonful of chia seeds (optional)

Two servings.

Steps:

1. Blend frozen pineapple, turmeric powder, grated ginger, banana, and coconut water.
2. Blend until smooth and creamy.
3. Pour into glasses and garnish with chia seeds, if preferred.
4. Serve immediately for a refreshing, anti-inflammatory breakfast.

Notes, Features, and Variations:

- Add a squeeze of lime juice for added flavor.
- Add a handful of spinach for extra nutrition.
- For added sweetness, sprinkle with honey or maple syrup.

Utensils needed: blender and cups.

Nutritional information:

Per serving: 180 calories, 3g protein, 1g fat, 45g carbohydrates, and 6g fiber.

Recipe #18: Mediterranean Egg Muffins

These Mediterranean Egg Muffins are a high-protein, flavorful breakfast alternative for those with gastritis. These muffins, filled with cherry tomatoes, spinach, and feta cheese, are not only delicious but also simple to make ahead of time for a quick breakfast.

Ingredients:

- 6 big eggs.
- 1 cup baby spinach,
- 1/2 cup cherry tomatoes,
- 1/4 cup crumbled feta cheese,
- 1/4 cup black olives.
- Salt and pepper to taste.

6 servings.

Steps

1. Preheat the oven to 350°F (175°C).
2. In a bowl, mix together the eggs and season with salt and pepper.
3. Add chopped spinach, diced tomatoes, feta cheese, and sliced olives.
4. Transfer the mixture to buttered muffin cups.
5. Bake for 15-20 minutes, or until the eggs have set.
6. Let the muffins cool slightly before removing from the cups.
7. Serve warm or refrigerate for later.

Notes, Features, and Variations:

- Add more veggies, such as bell peppers or onions.
- To change the taste profile, use goat cheese for feta cheese.
- These muffins may be kept in the fridge for up to three days.

Utensils needed are a muffin tray, whisk, and mixing bowl.

Nutritional information:

Per serving: 120 calories, 9g protein, 8g fat, 3g carbohydrates, and 1g fiber.

Recipe #19: Pumpkin Spice Oatmeal

Enjoy the scents of autumn with our Pumpkin Spice Oatmeal. This fiber-rich and warm breakfast choice blends the heartiness of oatmeal with the seasonal sweetness of pumpkin and fragrant spices. A cozy and gastritis-friendly option for a hearty breakfast meal.

Ingredient list:

- 1/2 cup rolled oats,
- 1 cup unsweetened almond milk.
- 1/4 cup canned pumpkin puree
- 1/2 teaspoon pumpkin spice blend.
- 1 tablespoon maple syrup
- - 1 tablespoon chopped pecans (optional).

Two servings.

Step 1: In a saucepan, mix rolled oats and almond milk.
2. Bring to a simmer over medium heat.
3. Mix in the pumpkin puree, pumpkin spice, and maple syrup.
4. Continue cooking until the oats are cooked and the mixture is creamy.
5. Spoon into dishes and garnish with chopped pecans, if preferred.
6. Serve warm for a comforting and gastritis-friendly breakfast.

Notes, Features, and Variations:
- Add a sprinkle of ground cinnamon for more flavor.
- Adjust the sweetness with a drizzle of honey or a sprinkling of brown sugar.
- Add dried cranberries or raisins for a punch of sweetness.

Utensils required: Saucepan and stirring spoon.

Nutritional information:
Per serving: 250 calories, 6g protein, 8g fat, 40g carbs, and 6g fiber.

Recipe 20: Avocado and Chickpea Toast.

This Avocado and Chickpea Toast will take your toast game to the next level. Creamy avocado works nicely with seasoned chickpeas, resulting in a protein- and nutrient-dense breakfast alternative. This flavorful and tasty meal is quick to prepare, making it ideal for hectic mornings.

Ingredients:

- 2 pieces of whole grain bread
- 1 ripe avocado.
- 1/2 cup canned chickpeas, washed, drained
- One tablespoon of olive oil.
- Lemon juice, salt, and pepper to taste.
- Optional toppings include cherry tomatoes and microgreens.

Two servings.

Step 1: Toast whole grain bread to desired crispiness.

2. In a bowl, combine mashed avocado, lemon juice, salt, and pepper.

3. In a separate dish, combine the chickpeas, olive oil, salt, and pepper.

4. Spread the mashed avocado evenly over each slice of bread.

5. Garnish with seasoned chickpeas.

6. Optional garnishes include cherry tomatoes and microgreens.

7. Serve immediately for a hearty and stomach-friendly breakfast.

Notes, Features, and Variations:

- Add a sprinkle of red pepper flakes for more spice.
- Experiment with different bread kinds, such as sourdough and whole grain.
- Drizzle with balsamic glaze for an additional layer of flavor.

Utensils needed are a toaster, mixing bowl, and spreading knife.

Nutritional information:

Per serving: 300 calories, 10g protein, 15g fat, 35g carbohydrates, and 8g fiber.

1: Grilled Salmon with Lemon and Dill.

Grilled salmon is not only tasty, but also easy on the stomach. This meal is high in omega-3 fatty acids and is ideal for individuals following a gastritis-friendly diet. The tangy lemon and fresh dill provide a rush of flavor without compromising health.

Ingredients:

- 4 salmon fillets,
- 2 tablespoons olive oil,
- 1 teaspoon lemon zest,
- 2 tablespoons fresh lemon juice.
- 2 tablespoons chopped fresh dill
- Salt and pepper to taste.

4 servings.

Step 1: Preheat the grill to medium-high heat.

2. In a small bowl, combine the olive oil, lemon zest, lemon juice, chopped dill, salt, and pepper.

3. Brush the salmon fillets with the prepared mixture.

4. Grill the salmon for 4-5 minutes on each side, or until it easily flaked with a fork.

5. Serve hot and sprinkle with extra dill if preferred.

Notes, Features, and Variations:

- For added flavor, marinate the salmon in the sauce for 30 minutes before cooking.

- This dish pairs well with a side of steamed vegetables or quinoa.

Utensils needed: Grill, basting brush, small dish.

Nutritional composition:

Per serving: - Calories: 250 - Protein: 30g - Healthy Fats: 14g - Omega-3 Fatty Acids: 1.5g

2. Roasted Turkey and Quinoa Stuffed Bell Peppers

These stuffed bell peppers are a gastritis-friendly alternative to traditional stuffed peppers. Packed with lean turkey and quinoa, this recipe offers a balanced and comforting meal while being easy on the stomach.

Ingredient list:
- 1 cup cooked quinoa
- 1 lb lean ground turkey
- 4 bell peppers, halved and seeds removed
- 1 cup diced tomatoes
- 1/2 cup black beans, drained and rinsed
- 1 teaspoon cumin - 1 teaspoon paprika
- Salt and pepper to taste
- 1/4 cup chopped fresh cilantro

4 servings.

Procedure:
1. Preheat the oven to 375°F (190°C).
2. In a skillet, cook ground turkey until browned. Drain excess fat.
3. In a large bowl, mix cooked quinoa, ground turkey, diced tomatoes, black beans, cumin, paprika, salt, and pepper.
4. Spoon the mixture into halved bell peppers.
5. Bake for 25-30 minutes until peppers are tender.
6. Garnish with fresh cilantro before serving.

Notes, Features, and Variations:
- Add a sprinkle of grated low-fat cheese on top before baking for extra indulgence.
- Use a variety of bell pepper colors for a visually appealing dish.

Utensils needed: Skillet, baking dish.

Nutritional composition: (per serving)
- Calories: 300 - Protein: 25g - Fiber: 6g - Vitamin C: 150% DV

3. Gingered Carrot Soup

Gingered Carrot Soup is a soothing and anti-inflammatory option for those with gastritis. Packed with nutrients, the natural sweetness of carrots combined with the warmth of ginger makes this soup both healing and delicious.

Ingredient list:

- 1 lb carrots, peeled and chopped
- 1 onion, chopped
- 2 tablespoons fresh ginger, grated
- 4 cups low-sodium vegetable broth
- 1 tablespoon olive oil
- Salt and pepper to taste
- Fresh cilantro for garnish

4 servings.

Procedure:

1. In a large pot, heat olive oil over medium heat. Add onions and sauté until translucent.
2. Add chopped carrots and grated ginger. Sauté for an additional 5 minutes.
3. Pour in the vegetable broth, bring to a boil, then reduce heat and simmer for 20-25 minutes until carrots are tender.
4. Use an immersion blender to puree the soup until smooth.
5. Season with salt and pepper to taste.
6. Garnish with fresh cilantro before serving.

Notes, Features, and Variations:

- Add a splash of coconut milk for a creamy texture. - This soup can be served hot or chilled, depending on preference.

Utensils needed: Large pot, immersion blender.

Nutritional composition: (per serving)

- Calories: 120 - Vitamin A: 400% DV - Vitamin C: 15% DV - Fiber: 4g

4. Baked Lemon Herb Chicken Thighs

Baked Lemon Herb Chicken Thighs are a gastritis-friendly delight, offering a burst of flavor without the need for heavy spices. This recipe is gentle on the stomach, making it an ideal choice for those seeking a soothing yet delicious meal.

Ingredient list:
- 4 bone-in, skin-on chicken thighs
- 2 tablespoons olive oil
- 1 lemon, juiced and zested
- 2 cloves garlic, minced
- 1 teaspoon dried thyme
- 1 teaspoon dried rosemary
- Add salt and pepper to taste.

4 servings.

Procedure:
1. Preheat the oven to 400°F (200°C).
2. In a bowl, mix olive oil, lemon juice, lemon zest, minced garlic, dried thyme, dried rosemary, salt, and pepper.
3. Place chicken thighs in a baking dish and brush with the prepared mixture.
4. Bake for 30-35 minutes or until chicken is golden brown and cooked through.
5. Serve hot, drizzling any remaining juices over the chicken.

Notes, Features, and Variations:
- For a citrusy twist, add orange juice and zest to the marinade.
- Pair with a side of roasted sweet potatoes or steamed broccoli.

Utensils needed: Baking dish, basting brush.

Nutritional composition: (per serving)
- Calories: 320 - Protein: 22g - Healthy Fats: 24g - Vitamin C: 20% DV

#5: Quinoa Salad with Cucumber and Mint

Quinoa Salad with Cucumber and Mint is a delicious and nutrient-dense dish that is simple to digest. This salad is high in protein and fiber, making it ideal for people trying to follow a gastritis-friendly diet without compromising flavor.

Ingredients:

- 1 cup cooked and cooled quinoa
- 1 diced cucumber
- 1/4 cup chopped fresh mint leaves
- 1/4 cup crumbled feta cheese
- 2 tablespoons olive oil
- 1 squeezed lemon
- Salt and pepper to taste.

4 servings.

Instructions:

1. In a large bowl, mix cooked quinoa, sliced cucumber, mint, and crumbled feta cheese.
2. In a small bowl, combine olive oil, lemon juice, salt, and pepper.
3. Pour the dressing over the quinoa and gently toss to incorporate.
4. Refrigerate for at least 30 minutes before serving to let the flavors to combine.

Notes, Features, and Variations:

- Add cherry tomatoes for additional color and freshness.
- This salad can be served on its own or as a side dish with grilled chicken or fish.

Utensils needed: Mixing bowl and whisk.

Nutritional Composition (per serving)

- Calories: 280 - Protein: 8 grams. - Fiber: 5 grams. - Healthy fats: 12g.

#6: Miso-Glazed Cod with Steamed Bok Choy

Miso-Glazed Cod with Steamed Bok Choy is a light and tasty dish that is gentle on the digestive system. The umami-rich miso sauce gives depth to the fish, while the steamed bok cabbage provides a light crunch. This meal is both tasty and helpful to individuals on the gastritis diet.

Ingredients:

- 4 cod fillets,
- 3 teaspoons white miso paste,
- 2 tablespoons mirin,
- 1 tablespoon soy sauce.
- 1 tablespoon honey,
- 1 teaspoon sesame oil,
- 4 baby bok choy (halved), and sesame seeds for decoration.

4 servings.

Step 1: Preheat the oven to 400°F (200°C).
2. In a mixing bowl, combine the miso paste, mirin, soy sauce, honey, and sesame oil to make the glaze.
3. Arrange the fish fillets on a baking sheet and brush with the miso glaze.
4. Bake for 15-20 minutes, or until the fish flaked easily with a fork.
5. Steam the bok choy for 5 minutes, until tender-crisp.
6. Place the fish on a bed of steaming bok cabbage and decorate with sesame seeds.

Notes, Features, and Variations:
- Marinate fish in miso glaze for 1 hour before baking to increase taste.
If you want, you may substitute spinach or kale for the young bok choy.

Utensils needed: Baking sheet, bowl, and steamer.

Nutritional Composition (per serving)
- Calorie: 220 - Protein: 25 grams. - Fiber: 3 grams. - Iron (10% DV)

#7: Butternut Squash and Sage Risotto

Butternut Squash and Sage Risotto is a rich and cozy recipe that is ideal for a gastritis diet. The gentle tastes of butternut squash and fragrant sage make this risotto both tasty and easy to digest.

Ingredient list:
- 1 cup Arborio rice,
- 2 cups diced butternut squash,
- 1 finely chopped onion,
- 2 teaspoons olive oil,
- 4 cups low-sodium vegetable broth (heated),
- 1/2 cup dry white wine (optional).
- 2 tablespoons chopped fresh sage,
- Salt and pepper to taste,
- Optional Parmesan cheese for decoration.

4 servings.

Steps
1. Sauté chopped onion in olive oil until transparent.
2. Add the Arborio rice and simmer for 2 minutes, stirring regularly.
3. Add the wine (if using) and simmer until mostly absorbed.
4. Gradually add the heated vegetable broth, one ladle at a time, stirring frequently.
5. Add the cubed butternut squash and keep adding stock until the rice is creamy and cooked.
6. Stir in the fresh sage, season with salt and pepper, and simmer for another 2 minutes.
7. Serve hot, possibly garnished with Parmesan cheese.

Notes, Features, and Variations:

- To increase creaminess, add a spoonful of Greek yogurt before serving.

- If preferred, use pumpkin or sweet potato instead of butternut squash.

Utensils needed: large pan and ladle.

Nutritional Composition (per serving)

Calories: 320. - Fiber: 5 grams. - Vitamin A: 200% DV. - Iron: 15% DV.

#8: Shrimp and Avocado Salad

Shrimp and Avocado Salad is a light and pleasant dinner that is suitable for those with gastritis. The mix of delicious shrimp, creamy avocado, and crisp veggies produces a filling dish that is easy on the stomach.

Ingredient list:
- 1 lb peeled and deveined shrimp,
- 2 diced avocados,
- 1 cup halved cherry tomatoes,
- 1 diced cucumber.
- 1/4 cup finely chopped red onion,
- 2 tablespoons chopped fresh cilantro,
- 2 tablespoons olive oil,
- 1 juiced lime,
- Salt and pepper to taste.

4 servings.

Directions:
1. Cook shrimp in a pan until pink and opaque.
2. In a large mixing bowl, add cooked shrimp, chopped avocado, cherry tomatoes, cucumber, red onion, and cilantro.
3. In a small bowl, combine olive oil, lime juice, salt, and pepper.
4. Drizzle the dressing over the salad and gently toss to mix.
5. Serve cold.

Notes, Features, and Variations:
- Add chili powder for a bit of heat.
- For extra freshness, serve the salad on a bed of mixed greens.

Utensils needed: Skillet and big bowl.

Nutritional Composition (per serving)
- Calories: 280 - Protein: 20 grams. - Healthy fats: 18 grams - Vitamin C: 35% DV.

#9: Lentil and Vegetable Stew

Lentil and Vegetable Stew is a substantial and nutrient-dense meal for those with gastritis. This stew is rich in fiber and plant-based protein, making it not just light on the stomach but also tasty and comforting.

Ingredients:

- 1 cup dry green or brown lentils, rinsed

- 1 chopped onion

- Two carrots, diced

- Two celery stalks, chopped

- 3 garlic cloves, minced

- One can (14 ounces) of chopped tomatoes

- 4 cups of low-sodium vegetable broth,

- 1 teaspoon cumin,

- 1 teaspoon smoky paprika.

- Salt and pepper to taste.

- Garnish with fresh parsley.

4 servings.

Steps:

1. Sauté chopped onion, carrots, and celery in a large saucepan until softened.
2. Combine the minced garlic, cumin, and smoked paprika. Cook for an additional two minutes.
3. Add in the veggie broth, chopped tomatoes, and rinsed lentils. Bring to a boil.
4. Reduce the heat, cover, and simmer for 25-30 minutes, or until the lentils are cooked.
5. Add salt and pepper to taste.
6. Sprinkle with fresh parsley before serving.

Notes, Features, and Variations:

- Add balsamic vinegar to enhance taste.

- Optional: Serve over cooked quinoa or brown rice.

Utensils required: Large pot.

Nutritional Composition (per serving)

- Calories: 280 - Protein: 18 grams. - Fiber: 10 grams. - Iron: 25% DV

#10: Lemon Herb Baked Chicken Breast

Lemon Herb Baked Chicken Breast is an easy and delectable choice for individuals on a gastritis-friendly diet. The mild marinade of lemon and herbs improves the chicken's inherent juiciness, resulting in a meal that is both easy on the stomach and tasty.

Ingredients:

- 4 boneless and skinless chicken breasts.
- 3 tablespoons olive oil
- 2 teaspoons fresh lemon juice.
- One teaspoon dried oregano.
- 1 teaspoon dry thyme,
- Salt and pepper to taste, and lemon slices for garnish.

4 servings.

Steps:

1. Preheat the oven to 375°F (190°C).
2. In a dish, combine the olive oil, lemon juice, dried oregano, dried thyme, salt, and pepper.
3. Place the chicken breasts on a baking tray and brush with marinade.
4. Bake for 25-30 minutes, or until the chicken has reached an internal temperature of 165°F (74°C).
5. Finish with lemon slices before serving.

Notes, Features, and Variations:

- Marinate chicken for several hours or overnight for enhanced taste.
- To finish the dish, serve with roasted veggies.

Utensils needed: Baking dish and basting brush.

Nutritional Composition (per serving)

- Calorie: 220 - Protein: 28 grams. - Healthy fats: 10 grams - Vitamin C: 10% DV.

#11: Spinach and Mushroom Quiche with Oat Crust

Spinach and Mushroom Quiche with Oat Crust is a healthier version of a popular meal. The nutrient-dense spinach and mushrooms make a delicious filling, and the oat crust provides a healthy touch. This meal is easy on the stomach and a welcome addition to your gastritis diet.

Ingredient List for the Crust:
- 1 cup rolled oats,
- 1/4 cup olive oil,
- 1/4 cup water.
- 1/2 teaspoon salt

For filling:
- 2 cups chopped fresh spinach,
- 1 cup sliced mushrooms,
- 1/2 diced onion.
- 4 eggs
- One cup of unsweetened almond milk (or other plant-based milk)
- Salt and pepper to taste.
- Optional: 1/4 cup grated Parmesan cheese.

6 servings.

Procedure: For the Crust

1. Preheat the oven to 350°F/175°C.
2. Blend rolled oats in a food processor until they have a flour-like consistency.
3. Combine olive oil, water, and salt. Blend until dough forms.
4. Press the mixture into a pie plate to form the crust.
5. Bake for 10-12 minutes, until the crust is brown.

For filling:

6. In a pan, cook the mushrooms and onions until cooked. Add the chopped spinach and simmer until wilted.
7. In a dish, combine the eggs, almond milk, salt, and pepper.
8. Pour the egg mixture onto the sautéed veggies in the pie shell.
9. Optional: Sprinkle Parmesan cheese over top.
10. Bake for 25–30 minutes, or until the quiche is set.

Notes, Features, and Variations:

- Replace almond milk with lactose-free milk for a lactose-free alternative.

- To improve the flavor, add a touch of nutmeg or herbs.

Utensils needed include a food processor, pie dish, and pan.

Nutritional Composition (per serving)

- Calorie: 220 - Protein: 10 grams. - Fiber: 4 grams. - Calcium: 15% DV.

#12: Mediterranean Chickpea Salad

Mediterranean Chickpea Salad is a colorful and tasty dish that fits wonderfully into a gastritis-friendly diet. This salad, packed with fiber-rich chickpeas, fresh veggies, and a spicy dressing, is both relaxing and energizing to the taste senses.

Ingredients:

- Two cans (15 oz each) of drained and washed chickpeas.
- 1 cucumber,
- 1/2 cup cherry tomatoes,
- finely cut 1/2 red onion,
- 1/4 cup sliced Kalamata olives,
- 1/4 cup crumbled feta cheese.
- 2 tablespoons fresh parsley, chopped

For dressing:

- 3 tablespoons olive oil,
- 2 tablespoons red wine vinegar,
- 1 teaspoon dried oregano.
- Salt and pepper to taste.

4 servings.

Procedure:

1. In a large mixing bowl, add chickpeas, cucumber, cherry tomatoes, red onion, olives, feta cheese, and parsley.
2. In a small mixing bowl, combine olive oil, red wine vinegar, dried oregano, salt, and pepper to make the dressing.
3. Pour the dressing over the salad and gently toss to mix.
4. Let the salad marinade for at least 15 minutes before serving.

Notes, Features, and Variations:

- Add chopped bell peppers for additional color and crunch.

- To add more nutrients, serve the salad over a bed of spinach or mixed greens.

Utensils needed: large bowl.

Nutritional Composition (per serving)
Calories: 320. - Protein: 12 grams. - Fiber: 10 grams. - Healthy fats: 15 grams

#13: Quinoa and Roasted Vegetable Buddha Bowl

Quinoa with Roasted Vegetable Buddha Bowl is a healthy and well-balanced lunch for those with gastritis. This bowl is packed with colorful roasted veggies, protein-rich quinoa, and a drizzle of tahini sauce, making for a fulfilling and peaceful dining experience.

Ingredients:
- 1 cup cooked quinoa,
- 1 peeled and diced sweet potato,
- 1 sliced zucchini,
- 1 sliced red bell pepper.
- One cup cherry tomatoes, halved
- Two teaspoons of olive oil.
- 1 teaspoon cumin and season with salt and pepper to taste.

For the tahini dressing:
- 3 tablespoons of tahini
- 2 teaspoons of lemon juice.
- 1 clove garlic, minced
- Water (to thin down the dressing).
- Add salt and pepper to taste.

4 servings.

Steps:
1. Preheat the oven to 400°F (200°C).
2. Toss the sweet potato, zucchini, red bell pepper, and cherry tomatoes with olive oil, cumin, salt, and pepper.
3. Roast the veggies in the oven for 25-30 minutes, until golden and soft.
4. In a dish, layer the Buddha bowls with cooked quinoa and roasted veggies.
5. In a separate small bowl, combine the tahini, lemon juice, chopped garlic, salt, and pepper. Add water to get the required consistency.
6. Drizzle the Buddha bowls with the tahini dressing before serving.

Notes, Features, and Variations:
- Add baby spinach or kale for more greens.
- Add a sprinkling of pumpkin seeds to the dish for extra crunch.

Utensils needed: baking sheet and bowls.

Nutritional Composition (per serving)
- Calories: 380 - Protein: 12 grams. - Fiber: 8 grams. - Healthy fats: 18 grams

14: Salmon and Vegetable Foil Packets

Salmon and Vegetable Foil Packets provide a fuss-free and gastritis-friendly supper. The foil packages lock in the spices, resulting in moist and tasty salmon served with colorful veggies. This dish is not only simple to make, but also mild on the stomach.

Ingredients:

- 4 salmon fillets
- 2 sliced zucchinis
- 1 cup cherry tomatoes (halved)
- 1 thinly sliced red onion
- 2 tablespoons olive oil
- 2 minced garlic cloves
- 1 teaspoon dried dill
- Salt and pepper to taste
- Lemon wedges for serving

4 servings.

Step 1: Preheat the oven to 400°F (200°C).

2. In a mixing dish, combine sliced zucchini, cherry tomatoes, and red onion with olive oil, minced garlic, dried dill, salt, and pepper.

3. Place each salmon fillet on a piece of foil and cover with the vegetable mixture.

4. Close the foil packages securely and bake for 20-25 minutes.

5. Add lemon wedges for an added punch of flavor.

Notes, Features, and Variations:

- Experiment with other herbs, like as thyme or rosemary, for unique tastes.
- Before wrapping the salmon in foil, sprinkle fresh lemon juice over it to enhance moisture.

Utensils needed: baking sheet and aluminum foil.

Nutritional Composition (per serving)

- Calories: 300. - Protein: 25 grams. - Healthy fats: 15 grams - Vitamin C: 40% DV.

#15: Ginger Turmeric Carrot Soup

Ginger Turmeric Carrot Soup is a relaxing and anti-inflammatory alternative for gastritis sufferers. This antioxidant-rich soup mixes the sweetness of carrots with the warmth of ginger and turmeric, bringing both comfort and healing.

Ingredients:

- 1 lb carrots (peeled and chopped)
- 1 onion (chopped)
- 2 tablespoons grated fresh ginger
- 1 teaspoon powdered turmeric
- 4 cups low sodium vegetable broth
- 1 tablespoon coconut oil
- Salt and pepper to taste.
- Garnish with fresh cilantro.

4 servings.

Step 1: Sauté chopped onion in coconut oil until transparent.

2. Combine the diced carrots, grated ginger, and ground turmeric. Sauté for another 5 minutes.

3. Add the vegetable broth, bring to a boil, then decrease heat and cook for 20-25 minutes, or until carrots are soft.

4. Using an immersion blender, purée the soup until smooth.

5. Add salt and pepper to taste.

6. Before serving, garnish with chopped fresh cilantro.

Notes, Features, and Variations:

- Add lemon juice for a zesty flavor.
- Top with a spoonful of Greek yogurt for extra richness.

Utensils required: Large pot and immersion blender.

Nutritional Composition (per serving)

Calories: 120. - Vitamin A: 400% DV. - Vitamin C: 15% DV. - Fiber: 4 grams.

#16: Quinoa and Black Bean Stuffed Peppers

Quinoa and Black Bean Stuffed Peppers are a filling and protein-rich choice for a gastritis-friendly diet. These colorful peppers are packed with quinoa, black beans, and Mexican-inspired seasonings, making them both healthful and tasty.

Ingredients:

- 4 halved bell peppers with seeds removed
- 1 cup cooked quinoa
- 1 can (15 oz) black beans, drained and rinsed
- 1 cup fresh or frozen corn kernels.
- 1 cup chopped tomatoes,
- 1 teaspoon ground cumin,
- 1 teaspoon chili powder.
- Salt and pepper.
- 1/2 cup shredded cheddar cheese (optional).

4 servings.

Step 1: Preheat the oven to 375°F (190°C).

2. In a bowl, combine the cooked quinoa, black beans, corn, diced tomatoes, ground cumin, chili powder, salt, and pepper.

3. Fill each bell pepper half with the quinoa-black bean mixture.

4. If wanted, add some shredded cheddar cheese on top.

5. Bake for 25–30 minutes, or until the peppers are soft.

6. Serve hot.

Notes, Features, and Variations:

- Add fresh salsa or guacamole for extra taste.
- If you like, you may use brown rice for quinoa.

Utensils required: Baking dish.

Nutritional Composition (per serving)

- Calories: 280 - Protein: 12 grams. - Fiber: 8 grams. - Vitamin C: 200% DV.

17: Turkey and Vegetable Stir-Fry with Brown Rice.

Turkey and Vegetable Stir-Fry with Brown Rice is a simple and healthy meal for those with gastritis. This stir-fry is packed with lean turkey, bright veggies, and fiber-rich brown rice, making it a balanced and fulfilling dinner.

Ingredient list:

- 1 pound ground turkey,
- 2 cups broccoli florets,
- 1 sliced red bell pepper,
- 1 sliced yellow bell pepper.
- 1 julienned carrot
- 3 tablespoons low-sodium soy sauce.
- 1 tablespoon sesame oil,
- 1 tablespoon chopped fresh ginger,
- 2 minced garlic cloves.
- Two cups cooked brown rice.

4 servings.

Procedure:

1. In a large pan or wok, cook the ground turkey over medium-high heat.
2. Combine the sliced bell peppers, julienned carrot, broccoli florets, chopped ginger, and minced garlic. Stir-fry the veggies for 5-7 minutes, or until soft and crisp.
3. In a small bowl, combine the soy sauce and sesame oil. Pour the sauce over the turkey and veggies and mix to incorporate.
4. Serve the stir-fry with prepared brown rice.

Notes, Features, and Variations:

- Customize veggies to suit personal preferences.
- Drizzle with Sriracha for extra spice.

Utensils required: skillet or wok.

Nutritional Composition (per serving)
Calories: 320. - Protein: 20 grams. - Fiber: 5 grams. - Iron: 10% DV

#18: Greek Yogurt and Berry Parfait

Greek Yogurt and Berry Parfait is a delicious and gastritis-friendly dessert or snack. The combination of creamy Greek yogurt, fresh berries, and a dash of honey results in a delightful treat that is easy on the stomach while offering a rush of natural sweetness.

Ingredients:
- 2 cups Greek yogurt.
- One cup of mixed berries (strawberries, blueberries, raspberries)
- 2 tablespoons honey
- 1/4 cup granola (optional for crunch).

Two servings.

1. To serve, layer Greek yogurt, berries, and honey in glasses or bowls.
2. Repeat the layers until the glasses are full.
3. Optionally, top with granola for texture.
4. Serve cold.

Notes, Features, and Variations:
- Lactose-free Greek yogurt is a suitable alternative for lactose intolerant individuals.
- Sprinkle with chia seeds for added fiber and omega-3 fatty acids.

Utensils required: Serving glasses or bowls.

Nutritional Composition (per serving)
- Calorie: 250 - Protein: 20 grams. - Fiber: 3 grams. - Calcium (20% DV)

#19: Oven-Baked Sweet Potato Fries

Oven-baked sweet potato fries are a tasty and filling alternative to regular fries. These fries are packed with vitamins and fiber and cooked to perfection, with a crispy outside and a soft, sweet center that is both gratifying and easy on the digestive system.

Ingredients:
- 2 big sweet potatoes (peeled and cut into fries).
- 2 tablespoons olive oil
- 1 teaspoon smoked paprika.
- One-half teaspoon garlic powder
- Salt and pepper to taste.
- Garnish with fresh parsley.

4 servings.

Step 1: Preheat the oven to 425°F (220°C).
2. In a bowl, combine sweet potato fries, olive oil, smoked paprika, garlic powder, salt, and pepper.
3. Arrange the fries in a single layer on a baking sheet.
4. Bake for 25-30 minutes, flipping halfway through, or until the fries are golden and crispy.
5. Sprinkle with fresh parsley before serving.

Notes, Features, and Variations:
- Pair with a side of Greek yogurt and lemon for dipping.
- Add a sprinkle of cinnamon for a sweet and savory taste.

Utensils required: Baking sheet.

Nutritional Composition (per serving)
- Calories: 180
- Fiber: 4 grams.
- Vitamin A: 400% DV.
- Vitamin C (20% DV)

#20: Avocado and Chickpea Salad Wraps

Avocado and Chickpea Salad Wraps are a filling and stomach-friendly alternative for a light lunch or snack. These wraps, packed with protein-rich chickpeas, creamy avocado, and a refreshing combination of veggies, provide a flavorful burst without creating discomfort.

Ingredient list:

- One can (15 oz) of chickpeas, Drain and rinse.
- Two Mash ripe avocados.
- 1/2 cup halved cherry tomatoes,
- 1/4 cup finely chopped red onion,
- 2 teaspoons chopped fresh cilantro,
- 1 tablespoon lime juice.
- Salt and pepper to taste. - Use whole-grain tortillas.

4 servings.

Instructions:

1. In a bowl, mix chickpeas, mashed avocados, cherry tomatoes, red onion, cilantro, lime juice, salt, and pepper.
2. Mix well, crushing some of the chickpeas for texture.
3. Heat the whole-grain tortillas in a dry skillet or microwave.
4. Spread the avocado and chickpea mixture on each tortilla.
5. Fold the sides and roll up to form a wrap.

Notes, Features, and Variations:

- For added flavor, sprinkle with cumin or chili powder.
- For additional freshness, mix with a handful of spinach or arugula.

Use a bowl, pan, or microwave to warm tortillas.

Nutritional Composition (per serving)
- Calories: 300. - Protein: 10 grams. - Fiber: 8 grams. - Healthy fats: 15 grams

CHAPTER 5: DINNER DELIGHTS
1. Recipe title: Quinoa and vegetable stir-fry.

This colorful and nutrient-dense stir-fry is not only tasty, but also easy on the stomach. Quinoa, a complete protein, is combined with a variety of colorful veggies to provide a filling and gastritis-friendly dinner. Stir-frying enables a quick and uncomplicated preparation while maintaining the nutritious content of the ingredients.

Ingredients:
- 1 cup washed quinoa.
- 2 cups mixed veggies (bell peppers, broccoli, carrots, zucchini)
- 2 tablespoons olive oil
- 2 minced garlic cloves
- 1 tablespoon low-sodium soy sauce.
- 1 tablespoon rice vinegar,
- 1 teaspoon grated ginger, and
- Salt & pepper to taste.

Number of servings: four

Procedure 1: Cook quinoa according per package instructions.

2. In a large pan, heat the olive oil over medium-high heat.

3. Sauté the minced garlic and grated ginger for 1-2 minutes, until aromatic.

4. Add the mixed veggies to the pan and stir-fry until soft yet crunchy.

5. Stir in the cooked quinoa, soy sauce, rice vinegar, salt, and pepper. Mix thoroughly.

6. Continue to cook for 3-4 minutes, or until everything is well cooked.

7. Serve warm and enjoy this simple stir-fry.

Notes, Features, and Variations:

- Add protein with lean chicken or tofu.

- Experiment with various veggies based on your particular preferences.

- Use low-sodium soy sauce to minimize sodium levels.

- Garnish with fresh herbs such as cilantro or parsley.

Utensils required are a large skillet, wooden spoon or spatula, quinoa saucepan, and grater.

Nutritional composition:

Calories: 250 per serving Protein: 8 grams. Carbs: 40 grams Fiber: 6 grams. Fat: 8g

2. Baked Salmon with Lemon and Dill

This baked salmon dish is easy on the stomach and high in omega-3 fatty acids, which are recognized for their anti-inflammatory effects. The mix of lemon and dill offers a blast of flavor while being light and easy to digest.

Ingredient list:
- 4 salmon fillets
- 2 Tbsp olive oil
- Thinly slice one lemon
- Chop two tablespoons of fresh dill
 - Season with salt and pepper to taste.

Number of servings: four

Procedure:
1. Preheat oven to 375°F (190°C).
2. Arrange the salmon fillets on a baking pan lined with parchment paper.
3. Drizzle the fillets with olive oil and season with salt and pepper.
4. Place lemon slices on top of the salmon and sprinkle with fresh dill.
5. Bake in a preheated oven for 15-20 minutes, or until the salmon flakes easily with a fork.
6. Serve over steamed veggies or a simple salad.

Notes, Features, and Variations:
- Add honey for a hint of sweetness.
- Replace dill with other fresh herbs, such as parsley or chives.
- Make sure the salmon is acquired from a reliable and sustainable seafood vendor.

Utensils needed include a baking sheet, parchment paper, knife, and chopping board.

Nutritional composition:
Calories: 300 per serving |Protein: 25 grams. |Carbohydrate: 0g|Fiber: 0 grams.|Fat: 20g

3. Gingered Carrot Soup.

This calming gingered carrot soup is ideal for people who suffer from gastritis. Carrots contain critical vitamins and minerals, while ginger aids digestion. This warm and filling dish makes a great comfortable dinner.

Ingredients:

- 1 pound peeled and chopped carrots
- 1 diced onion
- 2 tablespoons olive oil
- 2 inches grated fresh ginger
- 4 cups vegetable broth
- Salt and pepper to taste
- Optional garnish: fresh cilantro

Number of servings: six

Procedure:

1. Heat olive oil in a big saucepan over medium heat. Add the chopped onion and sauté until transparent.
2. Cook for 3-4 minutes, tossing in chopped carrots and grated ginger.
3. Add the vegetable broth, bring to a boil, then decrease the heat and simmer until the carrots are soft.
4. Using an immersion blender, purée the soup until smooth.
5. Add salt and pepper to taste.
6. Serve hot, topped with fresh cilantro if preferred.

Notes, Features, and Variations:

- Adjust ginger amount to own taste preferences.
- Before serving, add a dash of coconut milk for an extra creamy texture.
- Freeze leftovers for easy future dinners.

Utensils required include a large saucepan, immersion or standard blender, cutting board, and knife.

Nutritional composition:

Calories: 120 per serving |Protein: 2 grams.|Carbohydrate: 20g|Fiber: 5 grams.|Fat: 5g

4. Turkey and Quinoa Stuffed Bell Peppers.

These turkey and quinoa filled bell peppers are both healthy and gastritis-friendly, thanks to their lean protein and whole grain content. The bell peppers supply vitamin C, while the turkey and quinoa help to balance the meal.

Ingredients:

- 1 cup cooked quinoa,
- 1 pound ground turkey,
- 4 split and seeded bell peppers,
- 1 chopped onion.
- 2 garlic cloves, minced
- 1 can (14 ounces) chopped tomatoes, drained
- 1 teaspoon cumin and 1 teaspoon paprika.
- Salt and pepper to taste.
- Garnish with fresh parsley.

Number of servings: Eight halves

Procedure:

1. Preheat oven to 375°F (190°C).
2. Cook ground turkey in a pan over medium heat until golden. Sauté sliced onion and minced garlic until tender.
3. Mix in the cooked quinoa, diced tomatoes, cumin, paprika, salt, and pepper.
4. Fill each bell pepper half with the turkey-quinoa mixture.
5. Place the filled peppers on a baking sheet and bake for 25-30 minutes, or until they are soft.
6. Sprinkle with fresh parsley before serving.

Notes, Features, and Variations:

- Customize using your preferred herbs and spices.
- For a vegetarian version, substitute lean ground chicken or tofu instead of ground turkey.
- Drizzle with a yogurt-based sauce for extra richness.

Utensils needed: baking sheet, skillet, cutting board, and knife.

Nutritional composition: Calories: 220 per serving (stuffed pepper half). | Protein: 15 grams. |Carbohydrate: 20g|Fiber: 4 grams.| Fat: 9g

5. Oat and Banana Pancakes

Begin the day correctly with these nutritious oat and banana pancakes. These pancakes are easy to digest and low in added sugars, making them an ideal breakfast option for individuals on a gastritis diet.

Ingredient list:

- 1 cup rolled oats

- 2 ripe bananas (mashed)

- 2 eggs

- One teaspoon of baking powder.

-1/2 teaspoon cinnamon

- 1/4 cup almond milk (or your chosen milk)

- One teaspoon vanilla extract.

- Coconut oil for cooking.

Servings: 2-3 (about 8 pancakes)

Procedure:

1. In a blender, mix rolled oats, mashed bananas, eggs, baking powder, cinnamon, almond milk, and vanilla extract. Blend until smooth.
2. Heat a nonstick skillet over medium heat, then add a tiny quantity of coconut oil.
3. Pour a tiny quantity of batter onto the griddle to make pancakes.
4. Cook until bubbles appear on the surface, then turn and cook the other side until golden brown.
5. Repeat until all of the batter is utilized.
6. Top with fresh berries or a dollop of yogurt.

Notes, Features, and Variations: - Add nuts or seeds to the batter for more texture.

- Drizzle with honey or maple syrup if tolerated.

- Experiment with various fruit toppings.

Utensils needed:

Tools required: blender, nonstick skillet, and spatula.

Nutritional composition: Calories: 180 per serving (3 pancakes).

Protein: 6 grams. | Carbs: 30g |Fiber: 4 grams. | Fat: 4g

6. Spinach and Chickpea Salad

This nutritious spinach and chickpea salad is simple to digest. Chickpeas are a fantastic source of plant-based protein, and the combination of spinach, cherry tomatoes, and cucumbers provides a range of nutrients. The mild lemon vinaigrette complements the tastes without overpowering the digestive system.

Ingredient list:

- 2 cups baby spinach,
- 1 can (15 oz) drained and rinsed chickpeas,
- 1 cup split cherry tomatoes,
- 1 diced cucumber,
- 1/4 cup crumbled feta cheese (optional).
- 2 tablespoons olive oil,
- 1 tablespoon lemon juice,
- 1 teaspoon Dijon mustard,
- Salt and pepper to taste.

Number of servings: four

Procedure:

1. To prepare, mix baby spinach, chickpeas, cherry tomatoes, cucumber, and feta cheese (optional).
2. In a small mixing bowl, combine olive oil, lemon juice, Dijon mustard, salt, and pepper to make the vinaigrette.
3. Pour the vinaigrette over the salad and gently toss to coat.
4. Serve immediately or chill until ready to serve.

Notes, Features, and Variations:

- Add more veggies, such as red peppers or onions.
- For added protein, add grilled chicken or tofu.
- Make a large quantity and store in an airtight container for a quick and easy lunch.

Utensils required: - Large mixing bowl - Small bowl for dressing. - Whisk or fork.

Nutritional composition: 200 calories per serving.

Protein: 8 grams. | Carbohydrate: 22g | Fiber: 6 grams. | Fat: 10g

7. Sweet Potato and Ginger Soup.

This silky sweet potato and ginger soup is a soothing option for gastritis sufferers. Sweet potatoes, which are high in vitamins and antioxidants, provide as a soft basis, while ginger adds warmth and improves digestion. This soup is simple to make and pleasant to the stomach.

Ingredients:
- 2 big sweet potatoes (peeled and diced)
- 1 chopped onion
- 2 tablespoons olive oil
- 2 grated fresh ginger
- 4 cups vegetable broth
- 1/2 cup coconut milk
- Salt and pepper to taste.
- Garnish with chopped chives.

Number of servings: six

Procedure:
1. Heat olive oil in a big saucepan over medium heat. Add the chopped onion and sauté until transparent.
2. Cook for 3-4 minutes, tossing in chopped sweet potatoes and grated ginger.
3. Add the vegetable broth, bring to a boil, then decrease the heat and simmer until the sweet potatoes are cooked.
4. Using an immersion blender, purée the soup until smooth.
5. Stir in the coconut milk and season with salt and pepper to suit.
6. Serve hot, topped with chopped chives.

Notes, Features, and Variations:
- Adjust ginger amount to own taste preferences.
- For a lighter version, use almond milk instead of coconut milk.
- Finish with a dollop of Greek yogurt for extra richness.

Utensils required include a large saucepan, immersion or standard blender, cutting board, and knife.

Nutritional composition: Calories: 180 per serving | Protein: 3 grams. | Carbohydrate: 28 grams | Fiber: 5 grams. | Fat: 7g

8. Lemon Herb Grilled Chicken

This lemon herb grilled chicken meal combines lean protein with vivid flavors, making it an ideal addition to a gastritis-friendly diet. The marinade offers a burst of zesty brightness, and grilling produces a light and easily digestible meal.

Ingredient list:

- Four boneless and skinless chicken breasts
- 1/4 cup olive oil.
- Zest and juice from 1 lemon
- 2 garlic cloves, minced
- Chopped fresh rosemary and thyme (1 tablespoon each).
- Add salt and pepper to taste.

Number of servings: four

Procedure:

1. To prepare the marinade, combine olive oil, lemon zest, lemon juice, minced garlic, rosemary, thyme, salt, and pepper in a bowl.
2. Put the chicken breasts in a resealable plastic bag or shallow dish and pour the marinade over them. Ensure that the chicken is uniformly coated. Marinate in the refrigerator for a minimum of 30 minutes.
3. Preheat the grill to medium-high.
4. Remove the chicken from the marinade and grill for 6-8 minutes per side, or until well done.
5. Allow the chicken to rest for a few minutes before slicing.
6. Serve with a side of roasted veggies or quinoa salad.

Notes, Features, and Variations:

- If an outside grill is not available, use a grill pan instead.
- Replace rosemary and thyme with other fresh herbs such as oregano or parsley.
- For added freshness, serve with a little lemon vinaigrette.

Utensils required include a grill or grill pan, a mixing bowl, and a reusable plastic bag or shallow dish.

Nutritional composition: Calories per serving: 220 | Protein: 30 grams. | Carbs: 2g
Fiber: 0 grams. | Fat: 10g

9. Cucumber and Avocado Gazpacho.

This cool cucumber and avocado gazpacho can help you beat the heat while also soothing your tummy. This soup, packed with hydrating ingredients, is a pleasant and easy-to-digest alternative. Cucumber, avocado, and herbs make for a lovely taste profile.

Ingredients:

- 2 diced cucumbers,
- 1 diced avocado,
- 1/2 cup chopped cilantro,
- 1/4 cup chopped mint.
- two green onions, chopped
- 2 cups vegetable broth,
- 1 lime juice,
- Salt and pepper to taste.
- Optional garnish: Greek yogurt.

Number of servings: four

Instructions:

1. Blend diced cucumbers, avocado, cilantro, mint, green onions, vegetable broth, and lime juice.
2. Blend until smooth, adding additional vegetable broth as required to get the desired consistency.
3. Add salt and pepper to taste.
4. Refrigerate the gazpacho for a minimum of 2 hours before serving.
5. Serve chilled, topped with a dollop of Greek yogurt if preferred.

Notes, Features, and Variations:

- Adjust lime juice and herbs to personal taste preferences.
- To increase protein, mix in cooked shrimp or crab flesh.
- Serve with whole-grain crackers or a small salad to complete the meal.

Utensils needed:

- Blender, chopping board, and knife.

Nutritional composition: Calories: 160 per serving | Protein: 4 grams. | Carbohydrate: 12g | Fiber: 5 grams. | Fat: 11g

10. Egg and Vegetable Breakfast Wrap.

Start your morning with this filling egg and vegetable breakfast wrap. This wrap, which is high in protein, fiber, and essential nutrients, is gentle on the stomach and provides long-lasting energy. Customize the filling to your liking.

Ingredients:

- Four large, beaten eggs.
- 1 cup diced vegetables (e.g., bell peppers, spinach, mushrooms)
- 4 whole grain tortillas
- 1/2 cup halved cherry tomatoes,
- 1/4 cup crumbled feta cheese,
- 1 tablespoon olive oil.
- Salt and pepper to taste.
- Garnish with fresh parsley (optional).

Number of servings: four

Procedure:

1. Heat olive oil in a pan over medium heat. Add the diced vegetables and sauté until tender.
2. Pour the beaten eggs over the vegetables and scramble until thoroughly cooked.
3. Heat the whole-grain tortillas in a dry pan or microwave.
4. Distribute the egg and vegetable mixture among the tortillas.
5. Finish each wrap with cherry tomatoes, crumbled feta, salt, and pepper.
6. Garnish with fresh parsley if desired.
7. Fold the tortilla's sides over the filling to form a wrap.

Notes, Features, and Variations:

- Add avocado slices for a creamy texture.

- Experiment with various herbs and spices to add flavor.

- Make it gluten-free by using corn tortillas or another gluten-free option.

Utensils needed: - Skillet - Spatula - Chopping board and knife.

Nutritional composition: Calories: 280 per serving | Protein: 12g| Carbohydrate: 20g| Fiber: 4 grams. | Fat: 16g |

11. Grilled Vegetable and Quinoa Bowl

Indulge in a nutritious and stomach-friendly meal with this grilled vegetable and quinoa bowl. Packed with antioxidants and fiber, this dish is a delightful combination of colorful vegetables and protein-rich quinoa. The light lemon-herb dressing adds a burst of freshness without compromising on ease of digestion.

Ingredient list:
- 1 cup quinoa, cooked
- 2 zucchinis, sliced
- 1 red bell pepper, sliced
- 1 yellow bell pepper, sliced
- 1 cup cherry tomatoes, halved
- 1 tablespoon olive oil
- 1 teaspoon dried oregano
- Salt and pepper to taste
- Lemon wedges for serving

Number of servings: four

Procedure:
1. Preheat the grill or grill pan over medium-high heat.
2. In a bowl, toss zucchini, red bell pepper, yellow bell pepper, and cherry tomatoes with olive oil, dried oregano, salt, and pepper.
3. Grill the vegetables until they are tender and have grill marks.
4. In serving bowls, layer cooked quinoa and grilled vegetables.
5. Serve with lemon wedges for a fresh squeeze before enjoying.

Notes, Features, and Variations:

- Add grilled chicken or tofu for extra protein.

- Drizzle with a balsamic reduction for added flavor.

- Customize with your favorite herbs and spices.

Utensils needed: - Grill or grill pan - Mixing bowl - Serving bowls

Nutritional composition: Calories: 250 per serving | Protein: 8 grams. | Carbohydrate: 40 grams | Fiber: 7g | Fat: 7g |

12. Lentil and Vegetable Stew

Warm up with this hearty lentil and vegetable stew, perfect for those looking for a gastritis-friendly comfort meal. Packed with plant-based protein and fiber, this stew is gentle on the stomach and provides a satisfying and nourishing option.

Ingredient list:

- 1 cup dry green or brown lentils, rinsed
- 1 onion, diced
- 2 carrots, sliced
- 2 celery stalks, chopped
- 2 cloves garlic, minced
- 4 cups vegetable broth
- 1 can (14 oz) diced tomatoes, undrained
- 1 teaspoon cumin
- 1 teaspoon smoked paprika
- Salt and pepper to taste.
- Garnish with fresh parsley.

Number of servings: six

Procedure:

1. In a large pot, combine lentils, diced onion, sliced carrots, chopped celery, minced garlic, vegetable broth, diced tomatoes, cumin, smoked paprika, salt, and pepper.
2. Bring the mixture to a boil, then reduce heat and simmer for 25-30 minutes or until lentils and vegetables are tender.
3. Adjust seasoning as needed.
4. Serve hot, garnished with fresh parsley.

Notes, Features, and Variations:

- Add leafy greens like spinach or kale for an extra nutrient boost.
- Experiment with different herbs and spices for varied flavors.
- Freeze leftovers for quick and convenient future meals.

Utensils needed: - Large pot - Wooden spoon - Cutting board and knife

Nutritional composition: Calories per serving: 220 | Protein: 14g | Carbohydrates: 38g Fiber: 12g | Fat: 1g |

13. Salmon and Avocado Salad

Elevate your salad game with this refreshing salmon and avocado salad. Packed with omega-3 fatty acids and essential nutrients, this salad is not only gentle on the stomach but also a delicious and satisfying option for a gastritis-friendly diet.

Ingredient list:

- 2 salmon fillets, grilled or baked
- 4 cups mixed salad greens
- 1 avocado, sliced
- 1 cup cherry tomatoes, halved
- 1/4 cup red onion, thinly sliced
- 2 tablespoons olive oil
- 1 tablespoon balsamic vinegar
- 1 teaspoon Dijon mustard
- Salt and pepper to taste

Number of Servings: 2

Procedure:

1. In a large bowl, toss mixed salad greens, avocado slices, cherry tomatoes, and thinly sliced red onion.
2. Top the salad with grilled or baked salmon fillets.
3. In a small bowl, whisk together olive oil, balsamic vinegar, Dijon mustard, salt, and pepper to create the dressing.
4. Drizzle the dressing over the salad and toss gently to coat.
5. Serve immediately for a light and satisfying meal.

Notes, Features, and Variations:

- Add a sprinkle of toasted nuts or seeds for crunch.
- Substitute balsamic vinegar with lemon juice for a citrusy twist.
- Customize with your favorite salad toppings.

Utensils needed: - Mixing bowl - Small bowl for dressing - Tongs or salad servers

Nutritional composition: Calories: 320 per serving | Protein: 20g | Carbohydrates: 14g Fiber: 7g | Fat: 22g |

14. Turkey and Vegetable Skewers

Bring a burst of flavor to your plate with these grilled turkey and vegetable skewers. Lean turkey is paired with colorful vegetables, creating a visually appealing and gastritis-friendly dish. The combination of herbs and spices adds depth without overwhelming the digestive system.

Ingredient list:
- 1 pound turkey breast, cut into cubes
- 1 zucchini, sliced
- 1 bell pepper (any color), cut into chunks
- 1 red onion, cut into wedges
- Two teaspoons of olive oil.
- 1 teaspoon dried thyme
- 1 teaspoon paprika
- Salt and pepper to taste
- Wooden skewers, soaked in water

Number of servings: four

Procedure:
1. In a bowl, combine turkey cubes, sliced zucchini, bell pepper chunks, red onion wedges, olive oil, dried thyme, paprika, salt, and pepper. Toss to coat evenly.
2. Thread the marinated turkey and vegetables onto soaked wooden skewers.
3. Preheat the grill to medium-high.
4. Grill the skewers for 10-12 minutes, turning occasionally, until the turkey is cooked through and the vegetables are tender.
5. Serve hot, accompanied by a side of quinoa or a light salad.

Notes, Features, and Variations:

- Customize with your favorite vegetables.

- Use metal skewers for convenience.

- Serve with a side of tzatziki or yogurt-based dipping sauce.

Utensils needed:

- Grill or grill pan - Mixing bowl - Wooden skewers

Nutritional composition: Calories: 250 per serving | Protein: 30 grams. | Carbohydrates: 10g | Fiber: 3g | Fat: 10g

15. Blueberry and Almond Smoothie Bowl

Start your day with a burst of antioxidants and energy with this blueberry and almond smoothie bowl. This delightful bowl is not only easy on the stomach but also rich in vitamins, minerals, and healthy fats. Customize the toppings to suit your taste preferences.

Ingredient list:
- 1 cup frozen blueberries
- 1 ripe banana
- 1/2 cup almond milk
- 2 tablespoons almond butter
- 1 tablespoon chia seeds
- Toppings: Sliced almonds, fresh blueberries, granola

Number of Servings: 2

Procedure:
1. In a blender, combine frozen blueberries, ripe banana, almond milk, almond butter, and chia seeds.
2. Blend until smooth and creamy.
3. Pour the smoothie into bowls.
4. Top with sliced almonds, fresh blueberries, and granola.
5. Enjoy with a spoon for a nutritious and satisfying breakfast.

Notes, Features, and Variations:
- Experiment with different frozen fruits for variety.
- Add a drizzle of honey for sweetness if desired.
- Incorporate spinach or kale for an extra nutrient boost.

Utensils needed: - Blender - Bowl - Spoon

Nutritional composition: Calories: 300 per serving | Protein: 8 grams. | Carbohydrate: 40 grams | Fiber: 10g | Fat: 14g

16. Shrimp and Quinoa Salad with Lemon Vinaigrette

This light and refreshing shrimp and quinoa salad are perfect for a gastritis-friendly lunch or dinner. With succulent shrimp, fluffy quinoa, and a zesty lemon vinaigrette, this salad offers a delightful combination of flavors while being easy on the stomach.

Ingredient list:

- 1 cup quinoa, cooked
- 1 pound shrimp, peeled and deveined
- 1 cucumber, diced
- 1 cup cherry tomatoes, halved
- 1/4 cup red onion, finely chopped
- 2 tablespoons olive oil
- 1 tablespoon lemon juice
- 1 teaspoon Dijon mustard
- Salt and pepper to taste
- Fresh parsley for garnish

Number of servings: four

Procedure:

1. In a large bowl, combine cooked quinoa, shrimp, diced cucumber, cherry tomatoes, and chopped red onion.
2. In a small mixing bowl, combine olive oil, lemon juice, Dijon mustard, salt, and pepper to make the vinaigrette.
3. Pour the vinaigrette over the salad and gently toss to coat.
4. Garnish with fresh parsley and serve immediately.

Notes, Features, and Variations:

- Add avocado slices for a creamy texture.
- Substitute shrimp with grilled chicken or tofu.
- Customize with your favorite herbs and spices.

Utensils needed: - Mixing bowl - Small bowl for dressing - Tongs or salad servers

Nutritional composition: Calories: 280 per serving | Protein: 22g | Carbohydrates: 25g Fiber: 4 grams. | Fat: 10g

17. Baked Cod with Herb Crust

This baked cod with a flavorful herb crust is a gentle yet delicious option for those with gastritis. The combination of fresh herbs, lemon, and a light breadcrumb crust enhances the natural flavors of the cod while ensuring easy digestion.

Ingredient list:

- 4 cod fillets
- 2 tablespoons olive oil
- 1/2 cup breadcrumbs
- 2 tablespoons fresh parsley, chopped
- 1 tablespoon fresh dill, chopped
- 1 teaspoon lemon zest
- Salt and pepper to taste
- Lemon wedges for serving

Number of servings: four

Procedure:

1. Preheat the oven to 400°F (200°C).
2. Place cod fillets on a baking sheet lined with parchment paper.
3. In a bowl, combine olive oil, breadcrumbs, chopped parsley, chopped dill, lemon zest, salt, and pepper to create the herb crust.
4. Press the herb crust mixture onto the top of each cod fillet.
5. Bake in the preheated oven for 15-20 minutes or until the fish is cooked through and the crust is golden brown.
6. Serve with lemon wedges for a fresh squeeze.

Notes, Features, and Variations:

- Substitute cod with other mild white fish like haddock or tilapia.
- Use gluten-free breadcrumbs for a gluten-free alternative.
- Garnish with more fresh herbs before serving.

Utensils needed: - Baking sheet - Parchment paper - Mixing basin

Nutritional composition: Calories: 180 per serving | Protein: 25 grams. | Carbohydrates: 8g | Fiber: 1g | Fat: 6g

18. Quinoa and Black Bean Stuffed Peppers

These quinoa and black bean stuffed peppers offer a pleasant and nutritious choice for anyone following a gastritis-friendly diet. The mix of quinoa, black beans, and spices makes a tasty and readily digested filling, while the bright bell peppers give critical vitamins.

Ingredient list:
- 1 cup quinoa, cooked
- 1 can (15 oz) black beans, drained and rinsed
- 4 bell peppers, halved and seeds removed
- 1 cup corn kernels (fresh or frozen)
- 1 cup salsa
- 1 teaspoon cumin
- 1 teaspoon chili powder
- Salt and pepper to taste.
- Garnish with fresh cilantro.

Number of servings: four

Procedure:
1. Preheat the oven to 375°F (190°C).
2. In a bowl, add cooked quinoa, black beans, corn, salsa, cumin, chili powder, salt, and pepper.
3. Fill each bell pepper half with the quinoa-black bean mixture.
4. Place filled peppers on a baking sheet and bake for 25-30 minutes or until the peppers are cooked.
5. Garnish with fresh cilantro before serving.

Notes, Features, and Variations:
- Top with a dollop of Greek yogurt or avocado for smoothness.
- Add a sprinkling of shredded cheese for added taste.
- Experiment with different varieties of salsa for differing heat levels.

Utensils needed include a baking sheet, a mixing dish, and a spoon for stuffing peppers.

Nutritional composition: Calories per serving: 240 (1 stuffed pepper half).
Protein: 10 grams. | Carbs: 45g | Fiber: 8 grams. | Fat: 3g

19. Berry and Chia Seed Parfait.

Enjoy a delicious and fulfilling treat with this fruit and chia seed parfait. This parfait, which contains antioxidants, fiber, and omega-3 fatty acids from chia seeds, is a delicious and easy-to-digest alternative for a gastritis-friendly dessert or breakfast.

Ingredients:

- 1 cup mixed berries (strawberries, blueberries, raspberries)
- 1 cup Greek yogurt.
- Two teaspoons of chia seeds
- 1 tablespoon of honey or maple syrup.
- Granola for toppings (optional)

Two servings.

Directions:

1. In a dish, combine Greek yogurt, chia seeds, and honey or maple syrup. Allow the mixture to settle for at least 30 minutes or overnight to thicken with the chia seeds.
2. In serving glasses, combine the chia seed mixture and mixed berries.
3. Repeat the layers until the glasses are full.
4. Add granola if desired.
5. Serve chilled and enjoy this nutritious and tasty parfait.

Notes, Features, and Variations:

- Try other fruits and berries.
- For a crunchier texture, sprinkle with nuts or seeds.
- For a vegan version, use dairy-free yogurt.

Utensils needed:

- Mixing bowl and serving glasses.

Nutritional composition: Calories per serving: 220 | Protein: 12 grams. | Carbs: 30g
Fiber: 8 grams. | Fat: 6g

20. Butternut Squash and Sage Risotto

This butternut squash and sage risotto is a comfortable and tasty solution for folks with gastritis. Creamy Arborio rice is combined with roasted butternut squash, fragrant sage, and a dash of Parmesan cheese to provide a delightful and easily digestible meal.

Ingredient list:

- 1 cup Arborio rice,
- 2 cups diced and roasted butternut squash,
- 1 finely chopped onion,
- 2 minced garlic cloves.
- 4 cups vegetable broth, warmed
- 1/2 cup dry white wine (optional).
- 2 tablespoons olive oil,
- 1 tablespoon chopped fresh sage,
- 1/4 cup grated Parmesan cheese,
- Salt and pepper to taste.

Number of servings: four

Procedure:

1. Heat olive oil in a large pan over medium heat. Add the chopped onion and sauté until transparent.
2. Stir in the arborio rice and minced garlic for 1-2 minutes, or until the rice is gently toasted.
3. If using, add the white wine and whisk until largely absorbed.
4. Pour in the heated vegetable broth one ladle at a time, stirring frequently. Before proceeding with the next addition, wait until the previous one has been mostly absorbed.
5. When the rice is almost ready, add the roasted butternut squash and fresh sage.
6. Continue to add liquid until the rice is creamy and cooked to your preference.
7. Stir in the Parmesan cheese and season with salt and pepper.
8. Serve hot, topped with sage and Parmesan.

Notes, Features, and Variations:

- Replace veggie broth with chicken broth if desired.
- For an extra serving of greens, add a handful of fresh baby spinach.
- Finish with a dab of balsamic glaze for extra sweetness.

Utensils needed: - Large pan and ladle - Wooden Spoon

Nutritional composition: Calories: 300 per serving | Protein: 7 grams. | Carbs: 55g | Fiber: 5 grams. | Fat: 7g

CHAPTER 6: SNACK TIME
#1. Title: Baked Sweet Potato Chips

These crunchy Baked Sweet Potato Chips are a tasty alternative to typical potato chips. Sweet potatoes are high in fiber and minerals, making them a healthy snack option for individuals on a gastritis diet.

Ingredient list:
- 2 medium-sized sweet potatoes.
- 2 tablespoons olive oil
- 1 teaspoon paprika.
- 1/2 teaspoon sea salt
- 1/4 teaspoon black pepper.

4 servings.

Procedure:
1. Preheat the oven to 375°F (190°C) and prepare a baking sheet with parchment paper.
2. Cut the sweet potatoes thinly using a mandolin or a sharp knife.
3. In a large mixing bowl, combine the sweet potato slices, olive oil, paprika, salt, and black pepper until equally coated.
4. Place the slices in a single layer on the prepared baking sheet.
5. Bake for 15-20 minutes, turning the slices halfway through, or until the chips are golden and crisp.
6. Cool the chips for a few minutes before serving.

Notes, Features, and Variations:
- Try various seasonings like garlic powder or rosemary to enhance taste.
- For optimal freshness, store in an airtight container.
- Serve with plain yogurt or a mild dip.

Utensils needed include a baking sheet, parchment paper, and a mandoline or sharp knife.
- Large mixing bowl.

Nutritional composition:
Per serving: 120 calories, 2g protein, 3g fiber, 7g fat, and 14g carbohydrates.

#2 Title: Greek Yogurt Parfait with Berries

Enjoy this refreshing Greek Yogurt Parfait with Berries, a delicious blend of creamy yogurt, antioxidant-rich berries, and a hint of honey. This snack is not only soft on the stomach, but it also contains probiotics, which promote digestive health.

Ingredient list:

- One cup plain Greek yogurt.
- 1 cup mixed berries (strawberries, blueberries, raspberries)
- 2 tablespoons honey
- 1/4 cup granola (optional).

Two servings.

Procedure:

1. To serve, layer Greek yogurt, mixed berries, and sprinkle with honey.
2. Layer until the glass is full, then top with a sprinkling of granola if preferred.
3. Serve immediately and enjoy!

Notes, Features, and Variations:

- Try lactose-free yogurt for a milder choice.
- Try different fruits and nuts to provide variation.
- To adjust sweetness, add more or less honey to taste.

Utensils needed include serving glasses or bowls.

Nutritional composition:

Per serving: 220 calories, 12g protein, 4g fiber, 8g fat, and 28g carbohydrates.

#3 Title: Cucumber Avocado Roll-Ups

These Cucumber Avocado Roll-Ups are a light and refreshing snack that is ideal for individuals on a gastritis-friendly diet. They are simple to prepare and delicious to consume, thanks to the hydrating cucumber and creamy avocado.

Ingredient list:
- 1 big cucumber
- 1 ripe avocado.
- 1 tablespoon of fresh lemon juice.
- Salt and pepper to taste.
- Garnish with fresh dill.

4 servings.

Procedure:
1. Using a vegetable peeler or mandolin, slice the cucumber lengthwise into thin strips.
2. In a mixing bowl, mash the avocado and add fresh lemon juice, salt, and pepper.
3. Spread a thin coating of avocado mixture on each cucumber strip.
4. Roll the cucumber strips and fasten them with toothpicks.
5. Garnish with fresh dill and serve.

Notes, Features, and Variations:
- Add a sprinkle of chili flakes for a spicy boost.
- Experiment with other herbs, such as cilantro and mint.
- To add extra richness, serve with plain Greek yogurt on the side.

Utensils needed:
- Vegetable peeler or mandolin - Toothpicks.

Nutritional composition:
Per serving: Calories: 70. 1g of protein, 3g of fiber, 6g of fat, and 5g of carbohydrates.

#4: Quinoa and Vegetable Stuffed Bell Peppers.

These Quinoa and Vegetable Stuffed Bell Peppers are a filling and nutritious snack that is gentle on the stomach. They are a nutritious alternative for individuals following a gastritis-friendly diet, since they contain protein-rich quinoa and colorful veggies.

Ingredient list:
- Four bell peppers, any color
- 1 cup cooked quinoa,
- 1 cup diced zucchini,
- 1 cup cherry tomatoes (halved),
- 1/2 cup chopped spinach,
- 1/4 cup crumbled feta cheese.
- Two teaspoons of olive oil.
- One teaspoon dried oregano.
- Salt and pepper to taste.

4 servings.

Procedure:
1. Preheat the oven to 375°F (190°C).
2. Cut the tops of the bell peppers and remove the seeds and membranes.
3. In a bowl, mix the cooked quinoa, zucchini, cherry tomatoes, spinach, feta cheese, olive oil, dried oregano, salt, and pepper.
4. Stuff each bell pepper with the quinoa and veggie combination.
5. Place the filled peppers on a baking tray and bake for 25–30 minutes, or until soft.
6. Let them cool somewhat before serving.

Notes, Features, and Variations:

- Replace feta with a lactose-free cheese if necessary.

- For added protein, mix in chopped chicken or tofu.

- Drizzle with balsamic glaze before serving for extra taste.

Utensils required: - Baking dish.

Nutritional composition:

Per serving: 230 calories, 7g protein, 7g fiber, 10g fat, and 30g carbohydrates.

#5 Title: Chia Seed Pudding with Mango

Chia Seed Pudding with Mango is a delicious and healthy dessert that is ideal for a gastritis-friendly diet. It's a pleasant snack or dessert option since it's high in omega-3 fatty acids and has a natural sweetness from mango.

Ingredients:

- -1/4 cup chia seeds.
- 1 cup unsweetened almond milk
- 1 tablespoon maple syrup or honey.
- 1/2 teaspoon vanilla essence,
- 1 chopped ripe mango.

Two servings.

Directions:

1. In a dish, combine chia seeds, almond milk, maple syrup, and vanilla essence. Stir thoroughly and set aside for 5 minutes.
2. Stir the mixture again to break up any clumps of chia seeds, and chill for at least two hours, or overnight.
3. Before serving, stir the pudding to ensure it has a smooth consistency.
4. Pour the chia pudding into serving glasses or bowls and top with chopped mango.
5. Serve chilled, and enjoy!

Notes, Features, and Variations:

- Try various fruits, such as berries or kiwi.
- Add a sprinkling of chopped nuts for extra crunch.
- To adjust the sweetness, add more or less maple syrup or honey as desired.

Utensils needed:

- Mixing bowl - Serving glasses/bowls

Nutritional composition:

Per serving: 200 calories, 5g protein, 12g fiber, 10g fat, and 26g carbohydrates.

#6 Title: Zucchini Hummus Bites

Zucchini Hummus Bites are a delicious and easy-to-digest alternative to regular crackers. Zucchini serves as a hydrated basis, and hummus adds a creamy and protein-packed topping, making them a great snack for individuals following a gastritis diet.

Ingredients:

- 2 medium zucchinis (sliced into rounds)

- 1/2 cup hummus, homemade or store-bought.

- Sliced cherry tomatoes (for garnish).

- Fresh parsley, chopped (to garnish)

4 servings.

Procedure:

1. Place zucchini rounds on a serving tray or individual plates.

2. Spread a tiny quantity of hummus on each zucchini round.

3. Garnish with sliced cherry tomatoes and fresh parsley.

4. Serve immediately and savor the crisp, refreshing bits.

Notes, Features, and Variations:

- Try other hummus tastes, including roasted red pepper or garlic.

- Add a drizzle of olive oil for added richness.

- To add more flavor, sprinkle with paprika or cumin.

Utensils needed:

- Serving platters or plates.

Nutritional composition:

Per serving: 80 calories, 3g of protein, 3g of fiber, 5g of fat, and 7g of carbohydrates.

#7 Title: Salmon and Cucumber Roll-Ups

Salmon and Cucumber Roll-Ups are a protein-rich snack with a refreshing cucumber flavor. Salmon contains omega-3 fatty acids, making it a heart-healthy choice for a gastritis-friendly diet.

Ingredient list:
- Four slices of smoked salmon
- One cucumber, peeled into ribbons
- 1/4 cup cream cheese.
- Fresh dill for garnish.

Two servings.

Procedure:
1. Place the smoked salmon slices on a clean surface.
2. Spread a thin layer of cream cheese on each piece.
3. Place the cucumber ribbons on top of the cream cheese.
4. Roll the salmon slices into little bite-sized roll-ups.
5. Secure with toothpicks and sprinkle with fresh dill.
6. Serve chilled and enjoy the delectable blend of tastes.

Notes, Features, and Variations:
- Replace cream cheese with goat cheese for a tart touch.
- For added freshness, pour in some lemon juice.
- Pair with a serving of mixed greens for a full snack.

Utensils needed:
- Tooth picks

Nutritional composition:
Per serving: 120 calories, 10g protein, 1g fiber, 8g fat, and 2g carbohydrates.

#8 Title: Turmeric Spiced Popcorn

Turmeric Spiced Popcorn is a tasty and anti-inflammatory snack that is ideal for those with gastritis. Turmeric imparts a warm, earthy flavor while offering possible health benefits.

Ingredients:

- 1/2 cup popcorn kernels.
- 2 tablespoons coconut oil,
- 1 teaspoon ground turmeric,
- 1/2 teaspoon ground cumin, and
- 1/2 teaspoon smoked paprika.
- Salt to taste.

4 servings.

Procedure:

1. Pop the popcorn kernels using your favorite technique (air popper, stovetop, or microwave).
2. In a small saucepan, melt the coconut oil over low heat.
3. Mix in the ground turmeric, cumin, smoked paprika, and a touch of salt.
4. Drizzle the turmeric spice mixture over the popped popcorn and stir until evenly coated.
5. Let it cool somewhat before serving.

Notes, Features, and Variations:

- Sprinkle nutritional yeast for a cheese taste.
- Add a dash of cayenne pepper for a spicy bite.
- Keep in an airtight container for future pleasure.

Utensils needed:

- Small saucepan.

Nutritional composition:

Per serving: 120 calories, 2g protein, 4g fiber, 8g fat, and 13g carbohydrates.

#9 Title: Almond Butter Banana Bites

These Almond Butter Banana Bites are a simple yet delightful snack that combines the creamy texture of almond butter with the natural sweetness of bananas. They're packed with potassium and healthy fats, making them a healthful snack.

Ingredients:

- Two sliced bananas.

- 1/4 cup almond butter.

- Optional toppings include chia seeds or crumbled nuts.

Two servings.

Procedure

1. Apply a tiny quantity of almond butter to each banana round.

2. To add texture, sprinkle chia seeds or smashed nuts on top.

3. Place the banana bits on a tray or serving dish.

4. Serve immediately as a fast and tasty snack.

Notes, Features, and Variations:

- Use whatever nut or seed butter you choose.

- Drizzle with honey to provide more sweetness.

- Freeze for a pleasant frozen treat.

Utensils needed:

- A serving platter or dish.

Nutritional composition:

Per serving: 180 calories, 4g protein, 5g fiber, 10g fat, and 23g carbohydrates.

10 Title: Carrot and Ginger Soup Shooters

Carrot and Ginger Soup Shooters are a calming and nutrient-dense alternative for a gastritis-friendly snack. The combination of carrots and ginger delivers anti-inflammatory benefits while also making a tasty appetizer.

Ingredients:
- Peeled and sliced carrots
- Grated fresh ginger
- Diced onion
- Vegetable broth
- Olive oil
- Add salt and pepper to taste.
- Garnish with fresh cilantro.

4 servings.

Procedure:
1. Heat olive oil in a saucepan over medium heat. Add the chopped onions and sauté until transparent.
2. Combine the diced carrots, grated ginger, vegetable broth, salt, and pepper. Bring to a boil, then decrease the heat and simmer until the carrots are soft.
3. Let the mixture cool somewhat before mixing until smooth.
4. Transfer the soup to tiny shot glasses or serving cups.
5. Garnish with fresh cilantro and serve as a tasty soup shot.

Notes, Features, and Variations:
- Add a pinch of cayenne pepper for a spicy flavor.
- Finish with a dollop of Greek yogurt for extra richness.
- Serve warm or cold, according to your liking.

Utensils needed:
- Blender - Pot.

Nutritional composition:
Per serving: Calories: 80. Protein: 2g, fiber: 3g, fat: 4g, carbs: 10g

11. Title: Spinach and Feta Stuffed Mushrooms

Enjoy these Spinach and Feta Stuffed Mushrooms, a delicious blend of earthy mushrooms, nutrient-rich spinach, and tangy feta. This appetizer not only tastes great, but it also contains vitamins and minerals that are good for gastritis.

Ingredient list:

- 12 big mushrooms (stems removed),
- 1 cup chopped fresh spinach,
- 1/4 cup crumbled feta cheese,
- 2 minced garlic cloves.
- Two teaspoons of olive oil.
- Add salt and pepper to taste.
- Garnish with fresh parsley.

4 servings.

Procedure:

1. Preheat the oven to 375°F (190°C).
2. In a pan, heat the olive oil over medium heat. Add the minced garlic and cook until fragrant.
3. Add the chopped spinach and heat until wilted. Remove from heat.
4. In a bowl, mix the sautéed spinach and crumbled feta. Season with salt and pepper.
5. Fill each mushroom cap with the spinach-feta mixture.
6. Place the stuffed mushrooms on a baking sheet and bake for 15-20 minutes, until soft.
7. Sprinkle with fresh parsley before serving.

Notes, Features, and Variations:

- Use goat cheese instead of feta.
- For additional warmth, sprinkle with nutmeg.
- Serve with a side of Greek yogurt to dip.

Utensils needed:

- Baking sheets - Skillets

Nutritional composition:

Per serving: 90 calories, 4g protein, 2g fiber, 7g fat, and 5g carbohydrates.

12 Title: Apple and Almond Energy Bites.

These Apple and Almond Energy Bites, a balanced combination of delicious apples, crunchy almonds, and oats, will satisfy your snack desires. These no-bake snacks deliver a quick energy boost while remaining flavorful.

Ingredients:

- 1 cup rolled oats,
- 1/2 cup finely chopped almonds,
- 1/2 cup dried apple,
- 1/4 cup almond butter,
- 2 tablespoons honey,
- 1/2 teaspoon cinnamon.
- A pinch of salt.

12 servings.

Procedure:

1. To make the recipe, mix rolled oats, chopped almonds, dried apple, almond butter, honey, cinnamon, and a pinch of salt.
2. Mix the ingredients together until they form a sticky dough.
3. Using clean hands, form the mixture into small, bite-size balls.
4. Place the energy bites on a tray and refrigerate for at least 30 minutes until solid.
5. Keep in an airtight jar in the fridge.

Notes, Features, and Variations:

- Add chia seeds or flaxseeds for added nutritional value.
- Experiment with various nut butters, such as peanut and cashew.
- For extra texture, roll the bits in shredded coconut.

Utensils needed include a mixing bowl and a tray for refrigeration.

Nutritional composition:

Per serving (one energy bite): 80 calories, 3g protein, 2g fiber, 4g fat, and 9g carbohydrates.

#13 Title: Rice Cake with Avocado and Tomato

This Rice Cake with Avocado and Tomato makes for a simple yet tasty snack. The creamy avocado complements the freshness of the tomatoes, resulting in a light and healthy treat appropriate for a gastritis-friendly diet.

Ingredient list:

- Four rice cakes.

- Mash one ripe avocado and chop one cup cherry tomatoes.

- One tablespoon of lemon juice.

- Add salt and pepper to taste.

- Garnish with fresh basil leaves.

4 servings.

Procedure

1. Spread a liberal amount of mashed avocado on each rice cake.

2. In a bowl, combine the sliced cherry tomatoes, lemon juice, salt, and pepper.

3. Spoon the tomato mixture over the avocado-coated rice cakes.

4. Garnish with fresh basil leaves and serve immediately.

Notes, Features, and Variations:

- Sprinkle with red pepper flakes for a spicy kick.

- Use multigrain rice cakes to boost nutritional value.

- Drizzle with balsamic glaze for added taste.

Utensils needed:

- None

Nutritional composition:

Per serving: 120 calories, 2g protein, 3g fiber, 7g fat, and 14g carbohydrates.

#14 Title: Berry and Mint Infused Water

Stay hydrated and rejuvenated with Berry and Mint Infused Water. Infusing water with berries and mint provides a blast of natural flavor, making it a refreshing and hydrating alternative to sugary drinks.

Ingredient list:
- 1 cup mixed berries (strawberries, blueberries, raspberries)
- Fresh mint leaves.
- 1 finely sliced lemon
- 8 glasses of water.

4 servings.

Procedure:
1. In a large pitcher, blend mixed berries, mint leaves, and lemon slices.
2. Fill the pitcher with water and gently swirl.
3. Refrigerate for at least 2 hours to let the flavors to combine.
4. Serve the infused water over ice and enjoy the pleasant flavor.

Notes, Features, and Variations:
- Try other berry combinations.
- Add cucumber slices for a refreshing twist.
- Fill the pitcher with water throughout the day for ongoing enjoyment.

Utensils needed:
- Large pitcher.

Nutritional composition:
Per serving: calories: 0, protein: 0g, fiber: 0g, fat: 0g, carbohydrates: 0g.

#15 Title: Grilled Eggplant and Tomato Skewers

Grilled Eggplant and Tomato Skewers are a tasty and fulfilling appetizer that is simple to digest. The mix of eggplant and tomato yields a tasty delight ideal for people following a gastritis-friendly diet.

Ingredients:

- 1 medium eggplant, cubed
- 1 cup cherry tomatoes.
- Add 2 tablespoons olive oil
- 1 teaspoon dried oregano.
- Add salt and pepper to taste.
- Soak wooden skewers in water.

4 servings.

Procedure:

1. Preheat the grill or grill pan.
2. In a mixing dish, combine eggplant cubes and cherry tomatoes with olive oil, dried oregano, salt, and pepper.
3. Thread the eggplant cubes and cherry tomatoes on the moistened wooden skewers.
4. Grill the skewers for 8–10 minutes, rotating regularly, until the veggies are cooked.
5. Serve the cooked skewers warm.

Notes, Features, and Variations:

- Drizzle with balsamic reduction for more taste.
- For a distinct flavor, season with garlic powder or smoky paprika.
- Serve with a side of tzatziki to dip.

Utensils needed:

- Grill or grill pan.
Wooden skewers

Nutritional composition:

Per serving: Calories: 90. Protein: 2g, fiber: 4g, fat: 7g, and carbohydrates: 7g.

CHAPTER 7: BEVERAGES AND GASTRITIS
Recipe #1: Soothing Ginger Mint Tea

This pleasant tea blends ginger's digestive advantages with mint's calming characteristics, making it an excellent choice for anyone suffering from gastritis. Both substances have long been used to relieve stomach pain and improve overall digestive health.

Ingredients:

- 1 inch thinly sliced ginger

- 1 tablespoon fresh mint leaves

- 2 cups hot water

- 1 teaspoon honey (optional)

Two servings.

Procedure:

1. Place sliced ginger and mint leaves in a teapot.

2. Pour boiling water over the ingredients and allow it steep for 5-7 minutes.

3. Pour the tea into mugs and add honey if desired.

4. Drink the tea carefully and enjoy the calming benefits.

Notes, Features, and Variations:

- Adjust honey to taste or eliminate for sugar-free alternative.

- If fresh ginger is unavailable, ginger tea bags can be used instead.

- Experiment with various herbs, such as chamomile, for further relaxing effects.

Utensils required: Teapot, knife, chopping board, and strainer.

Nutritional composition:

Calories: 10 per serving (no honey) 0g fat, 2g carbs, and 0g protein.

Recipe #2: Creamy Banana Oat Smoothie

This smoothie is a pleasant and nourishing choice for individuals on a gastritis-friendly diet. It contains potassium from bananas as well as oats, which have calming effects.

Ingredient list:

- 2 ripe bananas,
- 1/2 cup old-fashioned oats,
- 1 cup plain yogurt.
- Add 1 tablespoon honey
- 1/2 teaspoon ground cinnamon.
- One cup almond milk.

Two servings.

Procedure:

1. Blend bananas, oats, yogurt, honey, cinnamon, and almond milk.
2. Blend until smooth and creamy.
3. Pour into cups and drink immediately.

Notes, Features, and Variations:

- Use lactose-free or non-dairy yogurt for a dairy-free alternative.
- To adjust the sweetness, add more or less honey to taste.
- Add a sprinkle of ground flaxseeds for extra fiber.

Utensils required: blender, measuring cup, knife, and chopping board.

Nutritional composition:

Calories: 250 per serving, 5g fat, 48g carbs, 7g protein.

Recipe #3: Quinoa and Vegetable Broth

This light and nutrient-dense soup with quinoa and veggies is a nutritious choice for those with gastritis. It's mild on the stomach and high in critical vitamins.

Ingredients:

- 1/2 cup quinoa, washed
- 4 cups vegetable broth,
- 1 diced carrot,
- 1 chopped celery stalk,
- 1 sliced zucchini,
- 1 cup spinach,
- 1 teaspoon olive oil.
- Add salt and pepper to taste.

4 servings.

Procedure:

1. Heat olive oil in a saucepan over medium heat.
2. Combine carrots, celery, and zucchini. Sauté for five minutes.
3. Pour in the veggie broth and heat to a boil.
4. Add the quinoa and simmer for 15-20 minutes until cooked.
5. Stir in the spinach, season with salt and pepper, and simmer until it wilts.
6. Serve warm.

Notes, Features, and Variations:

- Add your favorite veggies, such as bell peppers or peas.
- For an added burst of flavor, pour in more lemon juice.
- To make it heartier, add shredded chicken.

Utensils required: Pot, knife, chopping board, and stirring spoon.

Nutritional composition:

Calories: 150 per serving, 3g fat, 26g carbs, 6g protein.

Recipe #4: Baked Salmon with Lemon and Dill

This baked salmon dish, which is high in omega-3 fatty acids and gentle on the stomach, is ideal for people looking for a gastritis-friendly protein alternative.

Ingredient list:
- 2 salmon fillets,
- 1 sliced lemon,
- 2 tablespoons minced fresh dill,
- 1 tablespoon olive oil.
- Add salt and pepper to taste.

Two servings.

Procedure:

1. Preheat the oven to 375°F (190°C).
2. Arrange the salmon fillets on a baking pan lined with parchment paper.
3. Drizzle the fillets with olive oil and season with salt and pepper.
4. Garnish with lemon slices and fresh dill.
5. Bake for 15-20 minutes, or until the salmon flakes easily with a fork.
6. Serve with a side of steamed veggies.

Variations:

- Use thyme or rosemary instead of dill to change the taste.
- Before baking, add a dash of white wine for additional moisture.
- Grill the salmon to get a smokey taste.

Utensils needed include a baking sheet, parchment paper, knife, and chopping board.

Nutritional composition:

Each serving has 250 calories, 15g of fat, 2g of carbohydrates, and 25g of protein.

Recipe 5: Roasted Sweet Potato and Carrot Soup.

This roasted sweet potato and carrot soup, which is high in beta-carotene and fiber, is both nutritious and mild on the digestive system, making it an excellent choice for people with gastritis.

Ingredients:

- 2 sweet potatoes, cubed
- 3 carrots, peeled and diced
- 1 chopped onion.
- 2 garlic cloves, minced
- 4 cups veggie broth,
- 1 teaspoon ground cumin.
- 1/2 teaspoon of smoked paprika.
- Salt and pepper to taste.
- 2 tablespoons olive oil.

4 servings.

Procedure:

1. Preheat the oven to 400°F (200°C).
2. In a large mixing bowl, combine sweet potatoes, carrots, onion, and garlic with olive oil, cumin, paprika, salt, and pepper.
3. Place the veggies on a baking sheet and roast for 30 to 40 minutes, or until soft.
4. Place the roasted veggies in a saucepan, add the vegetable broth, and heat to a boil.
5. Using an immersion blender, purée the soup until smooth.
6. Adjust the spice and serve hot.

Notes, Features, and Variations:

- Garnish with Greek yogurt or pumpkin seeds.

- To achieve a creamy texture, add a dash of coconut milk.

- Try various spices, such as ginger, for an added kick.

Utensils needed include a baking sheet, immersion blender, saucepan, knife, and chopping board.

Nutritional composition:

Each serving has 180 calories, 7g of fat, 27g of carbohydrates, and 3g of protein.

Recipe #6: Ginger Turmeric Golden Milk

This warm and pleasant golden milk, known for its anti-inflammatory characteristics, is an ideal beverage for those suffering from gastritis. The combination of ginger and turmeric adds taste while also potentially improving health.

Ingredients:

- 2 cups unsweetened almond milk,
- 1 teaspoon ground turmeric,
- 1/2 teaspoon ground ginger,
- 1 tablespoon honey,
- 1/2 teaspoon vanilla essence.
- A pinch of black pepper (to increase turmeric absorption)

Two servings.

Procedure

1. Heat almond milk in a small saucepan over medium heat.
2. Whisk in the turmeric, ginger, honey, vanilla essence, and black pepper.
3. Cook until warmed but not boiling, stirring constantly.
4. Pour into cups and savour the golden sweetness.

Notes, Features, and Variations:

- Consider using non-dairy milk substitutes such as coconut or oat milk.
- Adjust the sweetness by using more or less honey.
- To add more taste, sprinkle ground cinnamon on top.

Utensils required: saucepan, whisk, and measuring spoon.

Nutritional composition:

Calories: 80 per serving, 3g fat, 14g carbs, 1g protein.

Recipe 7: Grilled Chicken with Avocado Salad

This grilled chicken and avocado salad, packed with lean protein and healthy fats, is a refreshing and stomach-friendly alternative for a full lunch.

Ingredient list:

- Two boneless, skinless chicken breasts.
- Two avocados, cut
- 4 cups mixed salad greens
- One cup cherry tomatoes, halved
- 1/4 cup balsamic vinaigrette dressing.
- Add salt and pepper to taste.

Two servings.

Procedure

1. Season chicken breasts with salt & pepper.

2. Grill the chicken until thoroughly done, about 6-8 minutes per side.

3. Slice the grilled chicken into strips.

4. In a large mixing bowl, add salad leaves, sliced avocado, cherry tomatoes, and grilled chicken.

5. Drizzle with balsamic vinaigrette and gently mix.

6. Serve immediately.

Notes, Features, and Variations:

- Add crumbled feta cheese for additional taste.

- Add your favorite homemade dressing for a customized touch.

- For an alternative protein, try grilled shrimp or tofu.

Utensils needed are a grill, tongs, knife, chopping board, and big bowl.

Nutritional composition:

Calories: 350 per serving, 20g of fat, 15g of carbohydrates, and 30g of protein.

Recipe #8: Berry and Chia Seed Parfait

This delectable parfait is not only a tasty treat, but it is also high in fiber and antioxidants. The mix of berries and chia seeds provides both nutritious value and a pleasant texture.

Ingredients:

- 1 cup mixed berries (strawberries, blueberries, raspberries)
- 1 cup Greek yogurt.
- Two teaspoons of chia seeds
- 1 tablespoon honey,
- 1/4 cup granola.

Two servings.

Instructions:

1. In a dish, combine Greek yogurt and chia seeds. Allow it to sit for 15 minutes so that the chia seeds may absorb the liquid.
2. In serving glasses or bowls, arrange the chia seed mixture, mixed berries, and granola.
3. Drizzle honey on top.
4. Repeat the layers until the glass is full.
5. Refrigerate for at least 30 minutes before serving.

Notes, Features, and Variations:

- Add flavored yogurt for more diversity.
- You may use maple syrup for honey if desired.
- Experiment with several varieties of granola to create different textures.

Utensils needed are a bowl, measuring cup, spoon, and serving glasses.

Nutritional composition:

Calories: 280 per serving, 10g fat, 35g carbohydrates, 15g protein.

Recipe 9: Cucumber-Mint Infused Water

Staying hydrated is critical for those with gastritis, and this cucumber mint flavored water provides a delicious twist to simple water. The cucumber promotes hydration, while the mint adds a mild taste boost.

Ingredients:

- 1 thinly sliced cucumber
- 1/4 cup fresh mint leaves.
- One lemon, thinly sliced
- Two quarts (8 cups). water
- Ice cubes (Optional)

4 servings.

Procedure:

1. In a large pitcher, mix cucumber, mint, and lemon slices.
2. Fill the pitcher with water.
3. Refrigerate for at least 2 hours to let the flavors to combine.
4. Optional: serve over ice.

Notes, Features, and Variations:

- Experiment with different citrus fruits, such as lime or orange.
- To release additional flavor, lightly crush the mint leaves before adding them.
- For a fizzy variant, mix with a dash of sparkling water.

Utensils required: Pitcher, knife, and cutting board

Nutritional composition:

Calories: 0 per serving; fat: 0g; carbohydrates: 0g; protein: 0g.

Recipe 10: Baked Turkey Meatballs and Zucchini Noodles

These baked turkey meatballs with zucchini noodles are a low-fat alternative to conventional meatballs, resulting in a tasty and fulfilling dinner that is perfect for a gastritis diet.

Ingredients:

- 1 pound ground turkey
- 1/2 cup breadcrumbs (gluten-free if desired)
- 1/4 cup grated Parmesan cheese and 1 egg.
- 2 garlic cloves, minced
- one teaspoon dried oregano.
- Season with salt and pepper to taste.
- Spiralize four medium zucchinis.
- One cup marinara sauce.

4 servings.

Procedure:

1. Preheat the oven to 375°F (190°C).
2. In a bowl, mix together the ground turkey, breadcrumbs, Parmesan cheese, egg, garlic, oregano, salt, and pepper.
3. Form the mixture into meatballs and place on a baking sheet.
4. Bake for 20 to 25 minutes, or until well done.
5. While the meatballs are baking, cook the spiralized zucchini in a skillet until just soft.
6. Heat the marinara sauce in a separate pan.
7. Place the turkey meatballs over the zucchini noodles and drizzle with marinara sauce.

Notes, Features, and Variations: - Optional: Use ground chicken or lean beef.

- Experiment with different herbs to create unique tastes.

- To garnish, sprinkle with fresh basil or parsley.

Utensils needed: baking sheet, bowl, spiralizer, pan, and spatula.

Nutritional composition:

Calories: 300 per serving, 15g of fat, 15g of carbohydrates, and 25g of protein.

Recipe 11: Coconut Rice Pudding with Mango.

This delicious coconut rice pudding with mango gives a sweet pleasure without deviating from a gastritis-friendly diet. Coconut milk provides a creamy texture, while mango gives a blast of tropical flavour.

Ingredients:

- 1 cup jasmine rice,
- 2 cups coconut milk,
- 1/4 cup honey,
- 1/2 teaspoon vanilla essence,
- Pinch of salt,
- 1 diced mango, and toasted coconut flakes for decoration.

4 servings.

Procedure:

1. Cook jasmine rice according to package instructions.
2. In a saucepan, mix cooked rice, coconut milk, honey, vanilla essence, and a bit of salt.
3. Simmer over low heat, stirring regularly, until the mixture thickens.
4. Once the rice pudding has reached the required consistency, remove from the heat and allow to cool.
5. Place the coconut rice pudding in dishes and top with chopped mango and toasted coconut flakes.

Notes, Features, and Variations:

- Use brown rice for more fiber.
- You may use maple syrup for honey if desired.
- For added warmth, sprinkle with cinnamon.

Utensils required: saucepan, spoon, and bowls.

Nutritional composition:

Calories: 300 per serving; fat: 15g; carbs: 40g; protein: 4g.

Recipe 12: Lentil & Vegetable Stew

This lentil and vegetable stew, which is high in plant-based protein and fiber, is a filling and healthy alternative for individuals following a gastritis-friendly diet. It's a filling dish that delivers necessary nutrients without skimping on flavor.

Ingredients:

- 1 cup dry green lentils, washed.
- 4 cups vegetable broth,
- 1 chopped onion,
- 2 sliced carrots,
- 2 chopped celery stalks.
- 2 garlic cloves, minced
- 1 teaspoon ground cumin
- 1 teaspoon smoked paprika.
- Salt and pepper to taste.
- 2 tablespoons olive oil.

4 servings.

Procedure:

1. Heat olive oil in a big saucepan over medium heat.
2. Combine the diced onion, carrots, celery, and garlic. Sauté until the veggies soften.
3. Mix in the lentils, vegetable broth, cumin, smoked paprika, salt, and pepper.
4. Bring the stew to a boil, then decrease the heat and simmer for 25-30 minutes, or until the lentils are cooked.
5. Adjust the spice as needed and serve hot.

Notes, Features, and Variations:

- Include leafy greens such as spinach or kale for added nourishment.
- Top with a dollop of Greek yogurt or a sprinkling of fresh herbs.
- Serve with brown rice or quinoa for extra texture.

Utensils required: Pot, knife, chopping board, and stirring spoon.

Nutritional composition:

Calories: 250 per serving, 7g fat, 35g carbohydrates, 15g protein.

Recipe 13: Lemon-Herb Baked Cod

This light and tasty lemon herb baked fish is a good choice for persons with gastritis who want a protein-rich lunch. The blend of herbs and citrus adds a burst of freshness without overloading the taste.

Ingredients:

- 2 cod fillets,
- 1 thinly sliced lemon,
- 2 tablespoons chopped fresh parsley,
- 1 tablespoon chopped fresh dill,
- 2 teaspoons olive oil.
- Salt and pepper to taste.

Serves: 2

Procedure:

1. Preheat the oven to 375°F (190°C).
2. Arrange the fish fillets on a baking pan lined with parchment paper.
3. Drizzle the fillets with olive oil and season with salt and pepper.
4. Garnish with lemon slices, fresh parsley, and dill.
5. Bake for 15-20 minutes, or until the fish flaked easily with a fork.
6. Serve over steamed veggies or a simple salad.

Notes, Features, and Variations:

- Consider using halibut or tilapia as alternative white fish.
- To enhance the flavor, add a dash of white wine or lemon juice.
- Experiment with other herb combinations, including thyme and chives.

Utensils needed include a baking sheet, parchment paper, knife, and chopping board.

Nutritional composition:

Each serving has 180 calories, 10g of fat, 2g of carbohydrates, and 20g of protein.

Recipe 14: Spinach and Feta Stuffed Bell Peppers

These spinach and feta filled bell peppers are a tasty and nutrient-dense solution for those with gastritis. The mix of veggies and feta cheese makes for a filling meal that is easy on the stomach.

Ingredients:

- 4 halved bell peppers with seeds removed
- 2 cups chopped fresh spinach
- 1 cup cooked quinoa
- 1/2 cup crumbled feta cheese
- 1/4 cup toasted pine nuts
- 2 cloves minced garlic
- One teaspoon dried oregano.
- Salt and pepper to taste.
- Use 2 tablespoons olive oil.

4 servings.

Procedure:

1. Preheat the oven to 375°F (190°C).
2. Warm the olive oil in a pan over medium heat. Add the minced garlic and cook until fragrant.
3. Add the chopped spinach and heat until wilted.
4. In a bowl, mix together the cooked spinach, quinoa, feta cheese, toasted pine nuts, dried oregano, salt, and pepper.
5. Fill each bell pepper half with the spinach-quinoa mixture.
6. Place the filled peppers on a baking sheet and bake for 25-30 minutes, or until they are cooked.
7. Serve warm.

Notes, Features, and Variations:

- Try brown rice instead of quinoa for a variation.
- For added freshness, add chopped cherry tomatoes to the stuffing mixture.
- Finish with a sprinkle of balsamic glaze before serving.

Utensils needed: Baking sheet, pan, knife, and chopping board.

Nutritional composition:

Calories: 220 per serving; fat: 12g; carbs: 22g; protein: 8g.

Recipe 15: Blueberry Almond Chia Pudding.

This blueberry almond chia pudding is a delicious and nutritious dessert or snack alternative. Chia seeds include omega-3 fatty acids and fiber, and blueberries offer natural sweetness and antioxidants.

Ingredients:
- 1/2 cup chia seeds,
- 2 cups almond milk,
- 1 tablespoon honey,
- 1/2 teaspoon almond extract,
- 1 cup fresh blueberries.
- Sliced almonds as garnish.

4 servings.

Directions:
1. In a dish, combine chia seeds, almond milk, honey, and almond essence.
2. Stir thoroughly and place in the refrigerator for at least allow 2 hours, or overnight, for the chia seeds to absorb the liquid.
3. Before serving, mix the pudding to ensure it has an equal consistency.
4. In serving glasses, layer the chia pudding with fresh blueberries.
5. Optionally, garnish with sliced almonds and an additional drizzle of honey.

Notes, Features, and Variations:
- Experiment with various fruits, such as strawberries and raspberries.
- Finish with a dollop of Greek yogurt for extra richness.
- For a chocolate twist, add a spoonful of unsweetened cocoa powder to the chia mixture.

Utensils needed are a bowl, measuring cup, spoon, and serving glasses.

Nutritional composition:
Calories: 180 per serving, 10g fat, 18g carbs, 5g protein.

Recipe 16: Turkey and Vegetable Stir-Fry

This simple and tasty turkey and vegetable stir-fry is a light and digestible meal for those with gastritis. It's a healthy and easy-to-digest dinner packed with lean protein and colorful veggies.

Ingredients:

- 1 pound ground turkey,
- 2 cups broccoli florets,
- 1 thinly sliced bell pepper,
- 1 julienned carrot,
- 2 minced garlic cloves.
- Two teaspoons of low-sodium soy sauce
- 1 tablespoon sesame oil,
- 1 teaspoon grated ginger,
- 1 tablespoon olive oil.
- Sesame seeds as garnish (optional)

4 servings.

Instructions:

1. Heat olive oil in a wok or big pan over medium-high.
2. Add the ground turkey and heat until browned.
3. Sauté garlic and ginger for 1-2 minutes.
4. Combine the broccoli, bell pepper, and carrot. Stir-fry the veggies for 5-7 minutes, or until soft and crisp.
5. Toss with soy sauce and sesame oil until well combined.
6. Optional: garnish with sesame seeds.
7. Serve with brown rice or quinoa.

Notes, Features, and Variations:

- Add your favorite veggies, such as snap peas or mushrooms.

- For a spicy kick, add a sprinkle of red pepper flakes.

- To change up the protein, substitute ground chicken or tofu.

Utensils needed are a wok or big pan, spatula, knife, and chopping board.

Nutritional composition:

Each serving has 280 calories, 15g of fat, 10g of carbohydrates, and 25g of protein.

Recipe #17: Mango Avocado Salsa

This colorful mango avocado salsa complements salads, grilled chicken, and seafood. The natural sweetness of mango and the smoothness of avocado give a pop of flavor to any dish without creating intestinal discomfort.

Ingredients: -

- Diced mango and avocado
- Finely chopped red onion
- Seeded and minced jalapeño.
- 1/4 cup fresh cilantro, chopped
- Juice from 1 lime
- Add salt and pepper to taste.

4 servings.

Instructions:

1. In a bowl, add diced mango, avocado, red onion, jalapeño, and cilantro.
2. Squeeze lime juice over the mixture and gently stir.
3. Add salt and pepper to taste.
4. Refrigerate for at least 30 minutes to let the flavors to combine.
5. Use as a topping on grilled foods or as a side salad.

Notes, Features, and Variations:

- Change the amount of spiciness by adding more or less jalapeño.
- Serve with tortilla chips for a delicious salsa dip.
- Try adding chopped tomatoes for added freshness.

Utensils needed: bowl, knife, and chopping board.

Nutritional composition:

Calories: 120 per serving; fat: 8g; carbs: 15g; protein: 2g.

Recipe 18: Quinoa and Black Bean Salad.

This protein-packed quinoa and black bean salad is simple to digest. It's a tasty and fulfilling alternative that features a range of bright veggies with a zesty lime dressing.

Ingredients:

- 1 cup cooked and cooled quinoa
- 1 can (15 oz) of drained and rinsed black beans
- 1 cup halved cherry tomatoes
- 1 cup fresh or frozen corn kernels.
- 1/2 red onion,
- 1/4 cup fresh cilantro, and squeeze 2 limes.
- 2 tbsp olive oil
- Season to taste with salt and pepper
- Optional garnish: avocado slices

4 servings.

Procedure:

1. In a large mixing bowl, add cooked quinoa, black beans, cherry tomatoes, corn, chopped red onion, and cilantro.
2. In a small mixing bowl, combine lime juice, olive oil, salt, and pepper to make the dressing.
3. Pour the dressing over the quinoa and gently toss to incorporate.
4. Refrigerate for at least 30 minutes to let the flavors to combine.
5. Optional: garnish with avocado slices before serving.

Notes, Features, and Variations:

- Add chopped bell peppers for more color and crunch.

- For added protein, add grilled chicken or shrimp.

- Serve as a side dish or eat it as a light supper.

Utensils needed: bowl, whisk, fork, knife, and cutting board.

Nutritional composition:

Each serving has 280 calories, 8g of fat, 42g of carbohydrates, and 10g of protein.

Recipe 19: Rosemary Lemon Baked Chicken Thighs.

These rosemary lemon roasted chicken thighs are a simple and tasty protein source that is suitable for those with gastritis. Aromatic rosemary and tangy lemon make for a wonderful variation on a classic recipe.

Ingredient list:
- Four bone-in chicken thighs with skin on
- 2 tablespoons olive oil
- 2 teaspoons chopped fresh rosemary.
- Zest and juice from 1 lemon
- 2 garlic cloves, minced
- Add salt and pepper to taste.

4 servings.

Procedure:
1. Preheat the oven to 400°F (200°C).
2. In a small bowl, combine olive oil, chopped rosemary, lemon zest, lemon juice, minced garlic, salt, and pepper.
3. Arrange the chicken thighs on a baking sheet lined with parchment paper.
4. Brush the chicken thighs with the rosemary lemon mixture, making sure they are thoroughly covered.
5. Bake for 30-35 minutes, or until the chicken has reached an internal temperature of 165°F (74°C).
6. Serve hot with your preferred side dishes.

Notes, Features, and Variations:
- Marinate chicken in rosemary lemon mixture for many hours for better flavor.
- Sprinkle with paprika for a mild smokiness.
- Before serving, garnish with more fresh rosemary and lemon wedges.

Utensils needed include a baking sheet, parchment paper, brush, small basin, knife, and cutting board.

Nutritional composition:
Each serving has 300 calories, 20g of fat, 1g of carbohydrates, and 25g of protein.

Recipe 20: Green Tea and Mint Infusion.

This green tea and mint infusion is a calming and hydrating beverage that is easy on the stomach. Green tea is recognized for its antioxidant benefits, while mint adds a pleasant touch to make a relaxing beverage.

Ingredient list:
- two green tea bags.
- 1 bunch fresh mint leaves,
- 4 cups boiling water.
- Agave syrup or honey (optional).

4 servings.

Instructions:
1. Combine green tea bags and fresh mint leaves in a teapot.
2. Pour boiling water over the teabags and mint leaves.
3. Allow it to soak for 3–5 minutes.
4. Remove the teabags and mint leaves.
5. Optional: sweeten with honey or agave syrup.
6. Pour into individual glasses and enjoy.

Notes, Features, and Variations:
- Adjust steeping time based on desired tea strength.
- Serve over ice for a pleasant iced tea alternative.
- Experiment with several varieties of mint, such as spearmint and peppermint.

Utensils required: teapot, cups, and spoon.

Nutritional composition:
Calories: 0 per serving (without sweetener); fat: 0g; carbohydrates: 0g; protein: 0g.

CHAPTER 8: DINING OUT WITH GASTRITIS

Dining out with gastritis may be a bearable and pleasurable event if approached correctly. This chapter offers practical recommendations for people with gastritis to navigate restaurant eating, make informed menu selections, and effectively convey their dietary demands to restaurant personnel.

Tips for Dining Out:

Eating out when treating gastritis necessitates careful preparation and alertness. Consider the following suggestions to make your eating experience more pleasurable and gastritis-friendly.

Plan Ahead:
- Check restaurant menus online for gastritis-friendly selections.
- Choose places that provide fresh, less processed products.

Timing:
- Choose off-peak meal hours to communicate with staff about dietary preferences.
- Instead of hurrying through meals, eat slowly to improve digestion.

Portion Control:
- Request lesser servings or share meals with dining mates to avoid overeating.
- Request a to-go container at the start of the dinner to lay aside any leftover portions.

- To avoid acidic and caffeinated beverages, go for herbal teas or lemon water.
- Limit your alcohol consumption, as it might irritate the stomach lining.

Listen to Your Body:
- Recognize your body's cues and stop eating when you feel full.
- Be mindful of trigger foods that may exacerbate your symptoms and avoid them.

Selecting Informed Menu Options:
Choosing gastritis-friendly alternatives from a menu needs some knowledge and awareness. Use these principles to make educated decisions.

Select Lean Proteins:

- Grill, bake, or steam lean proteins such as chicken, turkey, or fish.

- Avoid fried and strongly seasoned meats, since these may aggravate gastritis symptoms.

Embrace Whole Grains

- Choose whole grains such as brown rice, quinoa, or whole wheat pasta.

- Avoid foods with heavy cream-based sauces or excessive butter.

Vegetables:

- Add a variety of cooked or raw vegetables to your meals.

- Avoid acidic veggies such as tomatoes and instead go for milder choices like zucchini or carrots.

Mindful Fats:

- Choose healthy fats like olive oil, avocados, or almonds.

- Avoid fried and fatty foods, since they might cause discomfort.

Monitor Dairy Intake:

- If sensitive to dairy, go for lactose-free or low-lactose choices.

- Replace dairy-based dressings and sauces with alternatives such as vinaigrettes.

Communicating Dietary Needs with Restaurant Staff:

Clear communication with restaurant workers is essential for ensuring your dietary requirements are satisfied. When discussing your needs, use the tactics listed below:

Be Specific:

- Explain your dietary limitations and preferences to the server.
- Indicate whether you require changes to a meal, such as deleting particular components or altering cooking techniques.
- Ask questions regarding dish preparation procedures.
- Inquire about ingredient substitutions and alternate menu alternatives.

Mention Food Allergies:

- If you have food allergies in addition to gastritis, please notify the personnel.
- Emphasize the necessity of avoiding certain components to avoid allergic responses.

Request Customization:

- Request adjustments to match your dietary demands politely and assertively. Most restaurants are willing to meet unusual requests within certain limits.

Express Gratitude:

- Appreciate the staff's efforts to meet your dietary demands.
- Express gratitude for their help in making your meal experience pleasurable.

Beginning the path to better digestive health with the "Gastritis Diet Cookbook for Beginners" has been a step-by-step investigation of tasty, nourishing foods designed to calm and assist people with gastritis. As we conclude our culinary journey, it's critical to review the basic concepts of the gastritis diet and establish long-term recommendations for optimal gastritis care.

Recap on Gastritis Diet Principles:

1. Mindful Ingredient Selection: The gastritis diet prioritizes ingredient selection. The emphasis on complete, unprocessed meals high in vitamins, minerals, and antioxidants has been crucial. We investigated the advantages of lean proteins, whole grains, fruits, vegetables, and healthy fats to ensure that each dish is nutrient-dense and suitable for those with gastritis.

2. Fiber helps preserve intestinal health. The addition of fiber-rich meals such as fruits, vegetables, and whole grains promotes regular bowel movements, increases satiety, and improves overall gut health.

3. Maintaining a balance between fats and proteins is crucial. Choosing lean proteins and healthy fats, such as olive oil, avocados, and almonds, has supplied long-lasting energy without taxing the digestive system.

4. Hydration and Herbal Support: To ensure proper hydration, we recommend herbal teas and infused waters. Herbal additives such as ginger and mint have not only improved flavor but may also provide possible medicinal advantages for digestive ease.

5. Limiting Triggers: Throughout the cookbook, we've been mindful of potential trigger foods that might worsen gastric symptoms. We attempted to produce meals that nourish rather than irritate the digestive system by avoiding or limiting acidic, spicy, and excessively processed ingredients.

Long-term strategies for Gastritis Management:

1. Achieving a Sustainable Lifestyle: Beyond the recipes, living a gastritis-friendly lifestyle requires consistency and sustainability. Including these ideas in your everyday practice promotes a comprehensive approach to digestive health. As you progress, consider incorporating these dishes into your normal meal planning to make gastritis management a natural part of your routine.

2. Regular Monitoring and Adaptation: Gastritis is a dynamic condition with fluctuating symptoms over time. Regularly evaluating your food choices and their influence on your health is critical. Listen to your body, take note of any trends or triggers, and be prepared to adjust your diet accordingly.

3. Consultation with Healthcare Professionals: While this cookbook is a useful resource, it's crucial to consider specific health concerns. If you haven't already, consider working with healthcare specialists like dietitians or gastroenterologists to tailor your gastritis treatment strategy. They can offer specialized advise based on your specific health profile.

4. Holistic Wellness activities: In addition to food, holistic wellness activities play a key role in managing gastritis. Stress reduction measures, regular physical exercise, and appropriate sleep all play important roles in promoting overall health and intestinal harmony. Consider mindfulness, yoga, or meditation to supplement your nutritional efforts.

5. Establishing a Support System: Managing gastritis is not a lonesome experience. Create a support network that recognizes and promotes your dedication to digestive health. Share your gastritis-friendly dishes with friends and family to make eating a social and supportive experience.

Finally, the "Gastritis Diet Cookbook for Beginners" provides a starting point for anyone looking to adopt a gastritis-friendly lifestyle. It is more than just a collection of recipes; it is a tool for empowerment and understanding. As you appreciate the aromas of these recipes, may you discover not just gastronomic delight, but also a route to long-term digestive wellbeing. The concepts and tactics described on these pages are intended to be customizable, allowing you to construct a gastritis treatment plan that fits effortlessly into your life, guaranteeing a happy and long-term road to digestive health. Cheers to fueling your body, appreciating every mouthful, and creating a future of holistic wellbeing.